Fiction

A LITTLE UNSTEADILY INTO LIGHT

Edited by
Jan Carson
Jane Lugea

NEW ISLAND

A LITTLE UNSTEADILY INTO LIGHT
First published in 2022 by
New Island Books
Glenshesk House
10 Richview Office Park
Clonskeagh
Dublin D14 V8C4
Republic of Ireland
www.newisland.ie

Compilation and Introduction © Jan Carson, 2022
Compilation and Afterword © Jane Lugea, 2022

Individual stories © Respective authors, 2022

The rights of Jan Carson and Jane Lugea to be identified as the editors of this work
have been asserted in accordance with the provisions of the Copyright and Related
Rights Act, 2000.

Paperback ISBN: 978-1-84840-861-6
eBook ISBN: 978-1-84840-862-3

The epigraph is quoted from Erwin Mortier's *Stammered Songbook: A Mother's Book of
Hours*, translated from the Dutch by Paul Vincent (2015) and is reproduced by kind
permission of Pushkin Press.

British Library Cataloguing in Publication Data. A CIP catalogue record for this
book is available from the British Library.

Set in 11.5 on 14.2 pt Adobe Caslon Pro

Edited by Susan McKeever
Cover design by Luke Bird, lukebird.co.uk
Typeset by JVR Creative India
Printed by ScandBook, scandbook.com

New Island Books is a member of Publishing Ireland

10 9 8 7 6 4 5 4 3 2 1

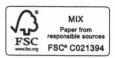

Contents

A human being is difficult poetry, which you must be able to listen to without always demanding clarification.

— Erwin Mortier

Introduction

Jan Carson

I was in my early twenties when my nana was diagnosed with dementia. She was the grandparent I was closest to. It wasn't just time spent together. In a family bent towards engineering and mathematics, Nana was my only fellow creative. She knitted the most incredible sweaters, making patterns up in her head. She sang and baked and played piano. She was deeply invested in the local community. Nana was the sort of person who didn't need to seek out stories. Stories seemed to cleave to her. As a fledgling writer I felt deeply at ease in her presence, chatting as we tootled about in her Mini Metro, or reading on her sofa while she played piano in the dining room.

It took almost a decade to lose my nana. At times this felt like a gradual erosion. The dementia slowly pared her back until she was barely recognisable; a much smaller woman, in every sense. There was a great deal of sadness in this journey but also moments of clarity, honesty and even joy. We laughed a lot. I had not anticipated laughter. However, subsequent experiences with dementia have taught me that humour can often be found in the odd situations it pitches you into. Dementia – much like life itself – isn't simple or easily defined. It's a muddle of competing emotions: the good, the bad and the ugly, often experienced simultaneously.

When Nana moved from her home to a residential care facility, she lost access to her beloved piano for the first time in seventy years of daily playing. The deprivation hit her hard. I could empathise. I knew I'd desperately miss reading and writing if these comforting practices were suddenly snatched away from me. It seemed like an unnecessary cruelty. Even now, nearly fifteen years into facilitating arts activities with older people, I still think about Nana and her absent piano each time I begin a new project. Every workshop is a fresh reminder that creativity and personal expression are part of what make us human. Everyone, including those living with dementia, has the right to access these experiences. Nana was my first significant encounter with dementia. I've had dozens, if not hundreds, since. Each has shaped me as both a writer and a human being. I've been challenged, frustrated, inspired and frequently humbled by the people I've met along the way.

There's a strong chance that you've been similarly impacted by dementia if you've chosen to pick up this book. I'm conscious that these stories may bring to mind a friend or family member who has dementia, or who you have lost to dementia. You may be living with dementia yourself. These stories will resonate on different levels depending upon your experience of the disease. There's no right or wrong reaction. We writers are just grateful for your consideration and time. Dementia is an umbrella term. It covers a wide range of diseases and conditions linked to memory impairment, difficulties with cognition and social ability. Each person living with a dementia will experience a unique set of symptoms and circumstances. No two dementia experiences are the same. Each fictional account of dementia in this book is equally unique. As you read the stories collected together in this anthology you may recognise situations and symptoms you're familiar with. You may also encounter a version of dementia radically different from the one you've experienced yourself. As the editor, I've actively sought out stories which explore a wide and eclectic range of dementia experiences. I wanted to reflect the full story of how dementia is impacting society.

It's almost impossible to estimate the true extent of dementia, however the Alzheimer's Society estimates that about 900,000 people in the UK have dementia at present. They expect this to rise to over 1 million by 2025. Whether you're a carer or family member, a neighbour, work colleague or friend, or you're living with dementia yourself, it's likely that the illness has already touched you or may soon become a significant part of your life. There are many reasons why dementia seems to be on the increase. A rise in life expectancy, better diagnosis rates and ongoing work to dispel stigma are all contributing factors. Dementia is not a new illness but society is slowly becoming more dementia aware. Organisations like Dementia NI and the Alzheimer's Society, which offer support and carry out vital research, have been active in promoting informed and positive messages about dementia. As a result, people living with dementia are much more empowered, vocal and visible than in the past. Though much work is still to be done in Ireland and the UK, and there are still some countries where people living with dementia are routinely hidden away or institutionalised, the practice of shaming or ignoring those living with dementia is thankfully on the decline.

These days, dementia is a topical subject, not least in the arts. Almost all the TV soaps have now included major storylines exploring dementia. Recent films like *Still Alice* and *The Father* have also tackled the subject, often to great critical acclaim. A contemporary explosion of memoir and non-fiction books shows there's not just an interest but also a market for writing which explores the reality of a dementia diagnosis. I'd thoroughly recommend reading some of these books. I've been particularly impressed with non-fiction works in translation by writers like Annie Ernaux, Arno Geiger and

Erwin Mortier, who has kindly given us the beautiful epigraph for this collection.

My own particular world is prose fiction – the reading, writing and dissecting of stories – and it's fair to say there's been a similar boom in dementia fiction over the last twenty years. In the last decade, all the major fiction prize lists have included novels like Avni Doshi's *Burnt Sugar* and Emma Healey's *Elizabeth is Missing* which explore the dementia experience. Pre-millennial prose writers occasionally included a character living with a dementia-like illness. Rarely was the condition named as such and, with a few notable exceptions, there were almost no novels entirely focused on dementia. Post-millennial writers appear much keener to consciously explore dementia in their fiction. This trend, though not without its problems, seems ripe for celebration and further study. It's heartening to see a growing number of academics around the world currently researching how dementia is depicted in contemporary writing, and constantly adding to the body of robust critical work on this important subject. Many of these academics have contributed to the collation of this anthology and I'm extremely grateful for their help.

I am not an academic. I'm a writer and arts practitioner. However, I jumped at the chance to join the ranks of academia for a couple of years. In early 2020, as the world geared up for a global pandemic, a small team of academics from Queen's University, Belfast began a research project funded by the Arts and Humanities Research Council, working with carers, trainee social workers, readers and people living with dementia to investigate how dementia is depicted in the words and thoughts of characters from contemporary novels. As a practising writer I was invited to join this project. My role was to ensure our research had a meaningful impact on the wider community. I took part in reading groups, discussing our ten key texts. I facilitated workshops for emerging writers who wished to wrestle with the ethics and practicalities of writing about dementia. I helped to run a first-of-its-kind symposium, bringing together academics, writers, support organisations and, most importantly, people living with dementia. We shared stories, frustrations and ideas. We discussed how to write well about dementia. It felt like the beginning of an incredibly significant conversation. I learnt an enormous amount in two short days.

Over the course of the project, I also read approximately one hundred fictional accounts of dementia. I read novels, stories and plays from across the world. I read books for children and young adults, crime fiction, magical realism, graphic novels, science fiction, literary fiction, romance and just about every other genre in existence. Some of the writing was truly brilliant and included deftly drawn characters whose dementia served to make them more believable and interesting. Some of the books I read were dire. They recycled tired tropes and lazy clichés. Some writers appeared to have done absolutely no research and as a result had written books which were at best factually inaccurate and at worst, downright dangerous. While it was encouraging to see more writers engaging with dementia, it was abundantly clear there was still room for improvement. I soon realised there was a distinct lack of diversity in the dementia novels and short stories which have so far emerged. This anthology of newly commissioned short stories is a small attempt to redress the existing balance of dementia fiction. The fourteen established and emerging writers included here have personal experience of the illness. They've brought their own diverse backgrounds to their writing. They've spent time in workshops discussing the ethics and practicalities of writing dementia. They've carried out significant research. In short, they've done their best to faithfully capture a lived experience which, though close, remains outside themselves. I believe that dementia offers the fiction writer a rare opportunity: a chance to think imaginatively and ethically about how we tell an other's story.

The question of appropriation currently looms large over literature. *Who owns a story? Can a story be owned? Is it wrong to write about something you have no lived experience of?* In the past, when a writer's creative integrity was questioned, they could simply cite the notion that fiction was 'just making stuff up' and from this, somewhat wobbly, platform continue to write from the perspective of whatever ethnicity, gender, class or sexual identity took their fancy, inventing experiences they were ignorant of. Thankfully most contemporary writers are much more aware of the harm and hurt which can be caused by the wilful or crass appropriation of someone else's story. However, there are still those occasions when writers find themselves drawn to another's stories which, for myriad reasons, have yet to be told, or moments when they'll wish to populate a novel with characters which aren't simply identikit versions of themselves. On such occasions an empathetic, ethical and creative understanding of how to write the unlived experience could provide a framework for avoiding the pitfalls commonly associated with appropriation.

There is a growing number of writers living with dementia who've written their own memoirs or collaborated to write in partnership. I'd recommend Wendy Mitchell's incredible books, written in partnership with Anna Wharton, and the work of Living Words UK who run bespoke writing projects for people with dementia. However, many people living with dementia will struggle to create a comprehensive and coherent narrative of their experience, particularly during the later stages of the illness. In compiling this anthology we've done our best to help the fiction writers we've included balance careful research with deep respect as they write about lives they have not lived, and experiences they've only been party to. A certain degree of careful appropriation is deemed necessary here, for if writers aren't willing to imagine the lived experience of dementia, many of these stories will never be told. The implications could be catastrophic. There's already a great deal of ignorance and fear surrounding dementia. Fear can keep people from seeking an early diagnosis and consequently rob them of the help and treatments available. The more dementia is represented diversely and honestly in the arts and media, the more the illness will be normalised and the less stigma those living with it will have to endure.

And yet, the writer's primary job is not to educate. The writers selected for this anthology had no remit to produce helpful, educational information, designed to help the reader better understand dementia. Fiction writers are first and foremost storytellers, lovers of language and makers of art. The commitment to telling a really good story has to override every other pressing agenda. All a writer of fiction is required to do is captivate and suspend disbelief. The fourteen pieces included in the anthology are, above all else, brilliant stories. They just happen to touch upon different aspects of dementia. They aren't bound by the need to put a positive or educational spin on the subject. A writer walks a fine line when fictionalising any big issue, be it dementia, the climate crisis or the latest scandal in Hollywood. The narrative is in constant tension with the desire to inform and interrogate. The writer's a bit like a lion tamer, holding the issue at bay in the corner so it isn't allowed to overwhelm the story, rendering it overly didactic, which is to say, a terrible read.

I've learnt the hard way that the trick to approaching a real-life issue like dementia from a fictional slant is to invest in great characters. Characters who are charged with depth and nuance. Characters who feel so real, the writer can simply take a back seat, allowing them to tell their own story in their own voice. If a character is simply a poorly developed mechanism for advancing the plot, the story itself will lack appeal and believability. In my reading research, I came across several examples of paint-by-numbers stock characters whose dementia felt like a rather obvious vehicle for adding an extra layer of confusion within a crime fiction plot or messing around with time and alternative realities in science fiction and magical realism. This isn't just bad dementia fiction. It's bad fiction full stop. Most great stories begin and end with interesting, complex and well-developed characters.

In this collection you'll meet intriguing characters you'll want to spend time with. You'll feel sympathetic and occasionally maddened and keen to discover more about their lives. You'll let these characters lead you into strange and sometimes difficult places because they are infinitely believable. If you're not careful, you might even forget for a moment that they and their stories are not real. Much has been written about the importance of fostering empathy in order to understand conditions like dementia. Extensive reading has taught me that an emphasis on character is perhaps the most essential facet of great dementia fiction. While an infographic or magazine ad can impart information, there's nothing like losing yourself in a character's world to begin the process of appreciating what a lived experience of dementia might feel like.

There is an increasing awareness of the need to offer people living with dementia support and community, often through peer-led groups. However, Wendy Mitchell, the writer and dementia activist, writes in her brilliant book, *What I Wish People Knew About Dementia*, 'In an ideal world, there wouldn't be any need for these niche groups. We only really have peer support groups because society won't make the adjustments that would allow us to integrate.' Much work still needs to be done but programmes like the Alzheimer's Society's fantastic dementia-friendly training scheme and other local and national-level projects have sought to make it easier for people living with dementia to integrate into our communities in a natural, inclusive way. If widespread understanding of dementia increases and prevailing stigmas continue to be challenged, there's no reason why the future won't see a decrease in specialised dementia-focused groups and a bent towards more comprehensive integration where existing services and activities become welcoming, inclusive environments so people with dementia can participate and contribute alongside their neighbours and peers.

In my reading, I began to notice a similar trend within dementia narratives. Many of the novels which I read were not primarily focused upon dementia, yet included peripheral characters and incidental plotlines where dementia was a theme. It's heartening to see contemporary writers beginning to rethink what a snapshot of diverse community could look like within the context of a novel. As society begins to develop a more inclusive attitude to dementia, people with dementia will become even more visible. In the same way that it's becoming much less common to see fictional portrayals of a society which doesn't include disability, ethnicity, gender, class and sexual diversity, the incidental depiction of dementia should hopefully become a common occurrence on stage, page and screen.

Similarly, we can hope to see a wider range of characters living with dementia. Anyone can develop dementia. It's not just an old person's illness. It pays no heed to class, gender or ethnicity. Nice people develop dementia. Horrible people can get it too. Consequently fictional characters with dementia should also be diverse. They should exhibit every kind of human trait and emotion, be party to every kind of experience – including the intellectual and sexual – and evoke a huge range of responses from the reader. In short, every character with dementia should be unique and distinct. It seems almost redundant to say this, but I feel compelled to. I've read over a hundred dementia narratives yet I've come across very little nuanced understanding of diversity within the dementia experience.

The typical character who's living with dementia in contemporary literature is white, middle/upper class and invariably a woman; usually of the doddery but sweet variety. These characters almost always evoke feelings of sympathy and occasionally pity. It's easy to feel sympathetic towards these stereotypical characters because, aside from the odd feisty or humorous outburst, they're pretty nice people. Picture a kindly, cardiganed grandma who occasionally muddles up her words. Nine times out of ten we encounter these characters in a residential care facility. Most have the ability to self-finance their care, though they'll inevitably have a partner, child or concerned friend anxious to ensure their loved one is well looked after as they approach the end of life. I'm not going to name and shame any fellow writers but there are a huge number of these lazy depictions of dementia circulating round our bookstores and libraries.

I find these portrayals quite frustrating. I've spent more than fifteen years working in older people's arts engagement. I've frequently encountered incredibly diverse experiences of dementia and an ongoing struggle to access affordable care. It's not to say the kindly grandma with dementia doesn't exist – my nana was a case in point – but the bigger picture of dementia is a much more diverse and complex one. Furthermore, I've come to resent the way the vast majority of characters living with dementia are written to elicit sympathy. They're almost always the victims in a story. They are passive, reduced and frequently written with the implicit understanding that their worth is tied up in their past. Now, I've met some lovely people with dementia and it was really easy to spend time with them. I've also worked with irritating, demanding and downright obnoxious people who have dementia. Sometimes these traits are symptoms of their diagnosis. Sometimes they were just difficult people who happened to develop dementia. It feels reductive, and possibly even discriminatory, to suggest a person living with dementia has to fit into a stereotype. It goes against everything I know about how complex human beings are and, though it should not require saying, people living with dementia are human beings too.

In this anthology you'll find heroes and villains, tricksters and saints, mothers, fathers, lovers, friends, people whose past has overshadowed their present and people who are making a huge impact on the world they currently find themselves in. Each one is unique. Each one is a complex mix of emotion and experience. These characters might have dementia, but dementia's only a small part of who they are. You may recognise some of these people and the way they behave from your own experience of dementia. Other characters may be unfamiliar or even a little unsettling. You might find yourself wondering what's going on and whether the writer in question has misrepresented the dementia experience. As you read, please bear in mind that every dementia is unique. Dementia is not limited to elderly people. Dementia isn't just forgetting or misplacing words. A dementia diagnosis can impact a person's moods and emotion, spatial awareness, physicality, senses, relationship and personality. Dementia can affect every aspect of life. I've tried to include stories which question perceived notions of what dementia is.

Most writers, myself included, relish the opportunity to be challenged by our work. We like to learn and develop as artists through the process of creating something new. The writers commissioned to produce new stories for this anthology have talked about how stimulating and inspiring they found the project. Unlike many regular writing commissions, this project included plenty of room for research and discussion in the development process. Our team facilitated workshops focused on how language could be used experimentally and creatively to capture something of the dementia experience. We shared reading recommendations, hosted discussions, and made our research findings available to all the writers involved. The thirteen writers included here along with myself developed these stories, mindful of the constraints associated with writing dementia. It was an absolute joy to see how they rose to this challenge. They've all worked extremely hard to achieve authenticity in how they've portrayed the thought life and dialogue of characters living with dementia. I suspect that they've been shaped by the process, on both an artistic and human level. Whether you're reading or writing it, an encounter with a good story almost always leaves you a little changed.

My own writing practice has been changed by my experiences with dementia. I've become intrigued by the various patterns, tics and language constraints associated with the illness. Early on, I began to see the creative possibility in telling a truth a little slant or finding a more roundabout, poetic way of conveying a misplaced or muddled sentiment. I've spent a lot of time listening to the people I work with and revelling in the way they use words in striking and unusual ways. In my own writing, I've played around with the linguistic possibilities presented by repetition, under-lexicalisation and malapropisms, (all common language issues associated with dementia). I've also noticed and utilised other frequently recurring aspects of the dementia experience, such as changes in sensory awareness, confusion and a more fluid awareness of time and space. Rather than finding these constraints restrictive, I've felt temporarily liberated from the limitations of traditional literary language and form. It's felt like being given licence to experiment and play. This is a sentiment echoed by many of the writers who've contributed here. You'll see, in these stories, just how much they've enjoyed exploring the potential of the dementia narrative. They're grateful for the opportunity to see the world from a slightly different perspective and discover new ways to story their words.

And yet, dementia remains a slippery subject to pin down in words. The experience of living with dementia is so varied and personal it cannot be captured definitively on the page.

In researching and developing this anthology we've constantly walked a very fine line, balancing an honest representation of an illness which can be extremely cruel and devastating and for which there's currently no cure, with the lived experience of the people we know who are living hopefully, tenaciously and as well as they can with dementia. It would be a disservice to these people to paint a picture of dementia which is entirely negative and yet, as writers, we must also strive for realism, honestly capturing the moments when dementia makes life feel unbearable.

Consequently, I've chosen a quote from Samuel Beckett's *Krapp's Last Tape* as the title for this anthology. In my reading, I came across few examples of writing which better explore the dementia experience than this short play. Beckett manages to authentically capture the humour, pathos, profundity and confusion of trying to hold onto an understanding of yourself as memory erodes and language unravels. It's a short, but devastatingly powerful play which includes the stage direction, 'a little unsteadily into light'. I found this a helpful and accurate summary of our attempts to strike that fragile balance when writing authentically about dementia. I think these words also say something powerful about living as well as possible with dementia. Arguably, they speak to us all. For aren't most human beings simply doing their best to move a little unsteadily into light?

This Small Giddy Life

Nuala O'Connor

'Is that plastic?' Imy taps a fingernail against the urn. 'Trust Mam to end up in a shitty pot.'

'It's brass. Painted.' I frown and rub my hand over the cold surface. 'That's what I ordered, anyway.'

The urn sits on my kitchen counter, the lid wedged shut; I take a knife from the block and prise it open. We peer in at the ashes.

'Wormy poo,' Imy says. 'Bird plop.'

'Cremains,' I say, and we both laugh, the same stupid, in-unison snorts we've done all our lives. I close the urn and it sits there, horribly present and, somehow, vital.

'What'll we do with her?' Imy asks.

'Same thing we always did with Mam, I suppose. Put up with her.' I sigh and push away tears with my fist. 'The last thing she got from me was blame, Imy.'

My sister shrugs. 'It doesn't matter, Sharon; she was beyond understanding, you said it yourself.' She pokes at the urn with the knife until I take it from her. 'What sort of blaming was it?' she asks.

I flick my hands through my hair and stare at the table instead of Imy. 'I said, "I've no clue how to fit into my own life, and it's your fucking fault, Mam." Do you think she heard? Understood?'

'She was hopped up on morphine, didn't even know where she was. Or who she was.'

I sigh. 'Well, none of us knew *that*.'

*

We move to a place where backstory is not allowed; over and again we move to this place. People are coldly civil towards my mother; she draws that out of them. Men like her well enough, but women are often hostile. Mam makes no pretence at being widowed, or still married to whomever, and she gets disapproval in return for her honesty, her lack of cover-up. God knows she hides everything else, but no one likes a woman alone in these places, especially one with two daughters. A handsome woman who might do harm to husbands; a woman who talks a lot, who asks questions, and reveals herself too soon. A woman with obvious appetites.

We move constantly because Mam is hunting down some elsewhere that will fit her and not one of these places is ever right. Up and down Ireland we drive, back and across: she needs to be near the sea; she needs the bustle of a town; she needs a friendly village; she needs the thrum of a big city; she needs a huge old house in the middle of a field, with only sheep for company. Nowhere works.

'There's something awful mean-spirited about Galway,' Mam says, after five months in Connemara.

Sligo is unmercifully wet.

Dublin frenetic and grey.

Villages are too native and small towns have no get-up-and-go.

On we travel.

In each new place, in the early days of our arrival, we sit in pubs while Mam cajoles information from landlords and locals.

'Would there be a little job going in here, by any chance?' she'll say, offering a lipsticked grin.

The barmen lean down, all silly smirks and bonhomie. 'Well, there just might be for a lassie like yourself. What's this you said your name was?'

'Margaret.' Wreaths of smiles. 'But my friends call me Meg.'

Mam asks barmen, too, about flats and houses, always determined to find something better than whatever shithole we've landed in 'for the time being'. But the time being is the only time our mother knows; there is no past, there is no planned-for future, those are inconveniences. In pub lounges all over the island, my sister and I sit at low tables, drinking cordial from glasses Laliqued with Tayto grease, while Mam perches at the bar, preens and flirt-chatters, and sips on a small stout, sweetened with blackcurrant.

Here we are in Ummoon, County Mayo. There we are in Portarlington, County Laois. Now we meet ourselves at the crossroads at Maam, blowing away from Clifden town as fast as we blew in. Meg driving and singing 'She'll be comin' 'round the mountain when she comes', or gripping the steering wheel in grim silence, which is worse. We don't know where we're from, Imy and I, or where we'll end up, and we don't dare ask our mother.

*

'You can get necklaces made with the cremains, you know,' I tell Imy. 'There's a website. They put the ashes into glass pendants. It looks like swirly sand.' I swizzle my finger in a circle.

Imy snorts. 'You want me to have Mam permanently around my neck? No fucking thanks, Sharon. Jesus, the things you come up with.'

'What? I thought it'd be nice. A bit of Meg to take back to Spain with you.'

'Nice! But why would you want to bother? The woman drove you mad.'

I frown. 'Not always, Imy. Her illness changed her; she wasn't as spiky as before.' I feel let down. 'And she was still our mother.'

*

I first notice a waywardness in Mam when she's turning sixty; she seems more harum-scarum than ever, yet more contained too. It's just small forgettings at first, and muddles about objects, about where exactly she lives.

She'll ask, 'Where's this I am now?'

'Galway,' I say. 'Rahoon. Remember? This is your flat.'

'Galway? Oh!' she replies, as if it's a curiosity to her.

She forgets, too, to keep her place clean, and she no longer asks anything about me: my daily doings, my job, my love life. These lapses begin to link together until I see something definite in her: a solid absence. It's as if she operates as two people: the reasonably together woman who knows me and acts like Mam, and the vague, incurious woman who appears when knowledge and truth are needed.

There's no sixtieth party planned for her – we've never gone in for celebrations – but Mam rings me the day before her birthday and demands that I come immediately to Rahoon, and I can tell she's agitated because she's lisping slightly and snapping out her words.

I grip my phone. 'What's wrong, Mam?'

'Just come over here, Sharon,' she barks, 'can't you do that for me?'

Life-things have kept me away from Mam's for a week and, when I let myself in, I'm stormed by a fruit-meat stink. Mam, though unruly in herself, has always preferred cleanliness. The bowl on the kitchen table – islanded in a sea of breadcrumbs – is packed with mildew-bloomy mandarins, and the draining board holds three opened tins of Whiskas, though my mother doesn't own a cat.

'The smell in here, Mam! Let me tidy up.' I tip the oranges into the bin.

She stalks up to me. 'That bitch at the bank won't let me have my money.' She's plucking at her hair with her fingers – a recent tic – her whole face rucked to a frown. 'I wanted a couple of grand for the party and that bitch says I can't have it. My own bloody money!'

I pull her hands gently away from her hair. 'What party, Mam?'

'My sixtieth, Sharon! For fuck's sake, what's wrong with you?'

'Oh. You never said you wanted a shindig. That's news to me.'

She squints at me as if I'm the worst kind of fool. 'It's all arranged.'

'But, Mam, you hate arranging things.'

'I do not. I booked the function room at the Spinnaker; I ordered a cake from O'Connor's,' she says.

'How?'

'I rang them.' Mam pauses. 'I went around there. To them. I walked to the bakery.' Her look to me is timid now, eye-slidey. 'And to the Spinnaker.'

I frown. 'And you're saying you walked all the way down to Salthill to book a function room?' She hardly ever leaves her flat. 'Are you sure about all this?'

Mam stalls. 'Imy organised it, actually,' she says, jutting her chin. 'I just need to pay now.'

'OK, but Imy's in Spain, so I don't see how–'

She holds her fingers to her temples. 'Stop, Sharon, stop! I need that money from the bank; you go there and talk to that wagon at the counter. The cheek of her! Everyone's coming to this party. Your father. Everyone.'

'My *father*?'

*

Mam lasts twenty-one months in Ennis, a long stint for us. The convent school accepts Imy and me, after a little histrionic wrangling with a sceptical nun.

'I'm a widow, Sister,' Mam says, squishing out a few tears.

The nun offers a brisk smile and nod, and we're in. Unlike other schools, I settle at the Mercy and make a friend called Emer, a fellow outcast. We bond because I'm a fatherless blow-in, and Emer's being raised by her grandparents, though her parents still live in the town. We walk home together after school and, in her company, I quit biting my nails to stumps, and sucking on my hair-ends. Emer means I can avoid home, avoid my mother and her tantrums.

Emer calls herself an ornithologist and, on our walks, she teaches me about bird habitats and behaviours, field-marks and feathers. We peer into bushes and treetops; we stake out fields and the riverbank.

'Always watch well, Sharon,' Emer instructs. 'Does the bird's tail fan? Does it wag?' She pats her chest. 'And look at the underbelly markings too. You need to be observant.'

We stalk every tree and bramble in Ennis.

'Do you want to see my collection of feathers?' Emer asks one day.

It's my first invitation to another girl's house and I feel sick with anticipation. Emer's grandparents are not the ancients I was expecting; they don't look much older than Mam. Emer's already whispered to me that her mother was fourteen having her – our age – and we've giggled and grimaced over the idea of letting a boy put his smelly thing inside our legs.

Her granny waves to us when we flit through the kitchen, to get to Emer's bedroom. There's a fireplace in the room and all along the mantelpiece are empty stout bottles, stuffed with feathers. I trail my fingers over the tops.

'Beautiful,' I say. 'They look like flames. Like flowers.'

'I really want to find kingfisher feathers; they're the prettiest of all the Irish birds. I'd love to see one – they fizz through the air.' She dive-zooms her hand.

'I'd love that too,' I say.

'Kingfishers foretell death,' Emer tells me, and I nod solemnly, as if this is something I already know.

'Have your tea here, Sharon. I'll get Granny to ring your mammy.'

Tea in Emer's house is egg sandwiches and cake, taken quietly around the kitchen table, on blue-striped plates. In our flat, it's foraged baked beans and toast, or whatever Imy and I can put together, while Mam works. Emer's granny and grandad butter slices of barmbrack and eat them without speaking. Nobody argues or accuses, shouts or rages, laughs or brings news, and I can barely swallow with the silence that echoes around my ears.

'I'll drive you home, Sharon,' Emer's grandad says, when we're finished.

I sit behind him in his car, my stomach trouncing with nerves, not knowing whether to speak. Do the Boyles *ever* talk? Do they fight? How do they know what each other thinks?

Emer's grandad insists on coming up to our flat above the butcher's shop, with its linger of lard and blood in the stairwell.

'I'm home,' I call, and Mam comes out to the corridor.

She taps her hand across her hair. 'Oh, Mr Boyle. Come in, come in.'

He follows her into the living-room, and I go to my bedroom, leaving the door ajar so I can spy. They talk for a minute about school, and Emer and me, then Mr Boyle steps close to Mam.

'If you ever need anything, Meg, just ask,' he says, 'anything now. I know a woman alone must face hardships.' His tongue pokes out like corned beef and he half-smiles. 'Anything you need at all.' He puts his hand on Mam's shoulder, then slides it down and squeezes her breast.

Mam jumps backwards. 'Well that I *don't* need,' she hisses.

Emer's grandad leaps, grabs his hat, and runs for the door. Though my cheeks are blazing, I muster nonchalance and come into the living-room. 'Is he gone?'

'Gone and good riddance, the old git,' Mam says. She looks angry, but she bursts out laughing and holds out her arms to me, and I run into them. She speaks into my hair, 'Don't let men undermine you, Sharon. Ever. Don't let them use and abuse you. Ever ever. Will you promise me that?'

I look up into her face. 'I promise, Mam.'

*

I hang birdfeeders like socks on a clothesline in Mam's yard. She sits inside at the window – a child new to television – following, in wonder, the finches and robins that plunder the nuts and seeds. I put a bird-spotting book on the windowsill beside her.

'I don't need a guide, the names are in here,' she says, tapping her forehead.

'Are they now?' I murmur.

Names and memories, places and history have flown from her head, with no will to return, it seems. The most ordinary things are alien to her now, as if they come as news. Vacancy possesses her, and I often find her stock-still and glassy-eyed, as if she has forgotten entirely who or where she is, and none of it matters, anyway. Where does her mind flee to in those arrested moments? What's behind the blank stare? I feel tender towards her when I notice she's gone, everything of who she once was slipped off into some other ether. All her travelling come to a dead stop.

*

Emer and I tramp through fields to the River Fergus and sit on the bank. A mallard streaks up and down in the water and we enjoy his emerald-headed majesty.

'Ducks are dabblers,' Emer says.

'Dabblers,' I repeat. She shifts her gaze and points to the sky; obediently, I look up. 'What is it?' I ask.

'Sparrowhawk.'

'Yellow eyes, rounded wings,' I offer. 'A sprinter.'

'Very good, Sharon.' I glimmer inwardly and we watch the sky until the hawk disappears. She shifts on the grass beside me. 'I saw you in town the other day.'

'Oh? I would've said hello if I saw you.'

'Myself and Granny were in a café, and I looked out, and there you were – you, your sister, and your mam.' She pinches my knee. 'She's like a film star, your mammy, you never said.'

I wince. 'Sure, why would I say that? She's just Mam.' I feel embarrassed. 'Imy calls her Mad Meg.' I snigger and Emer swings her head to glare at me. 'What?' I say.

'I'd smother my gran if it meant I could live with my mammy, that's the God's honest truth, Sharon. You don't know how lucky you are.' I nod solemnly and, when I see that she's crying, I squeeze her hand because I don't know what to say. 'My mam's gorgeous as well,' Emer says. 'She really is. But Granny always says "pretty women breed chaos". Do you think that's true?'

My cheeks flare and bars of iron run across my shoulders. I don't like Emer for saying this, but maybe that means it's the truth. *Chaos. Pretty women.* Is Mam chaotic? A bit, yes, I suppose, she can never settle, and she gets ragey about tiny things. Is she pretty? Certainly. Her dark hair makes porcelain of her skin, and she wears clothes like a shop mannequin, though they're all from charity shops. *Chaos?* Is it chaotic that Mam lashes out at us sometimes, when she's jarred? I can brazen up to her, so none of the slaps hurt; I puff out my cheeks when she goes at my face. Imy does the same. Mam's always sorry after, and she'll sleep in one of our beds, snotting and sobbing into our hair, saying, 'Never again, my little darling, never again.' But there's always an again.

I toss my head to loosen my thoughts. I glance at Emer and sniff deep. There's a dirty copper smell to the air and it sits heavily above us. I jump up.

'It's going to lash rain. I have to go,' I say, and I start to run.

I need to get as far away as I can from Emer and her remarks and her easy tears and her weird family and her bloody stupid birds.

*

I ring Imy from Mam's flat.

'You're there again?' Imy says, a small bit incredulous.

'I have to be. She forgets to eat. I need to make sure there's food inside her.'

'Like she always did for us?' Imy sniffs, and her stock of disgruntlements and grudges seems to make the line vibrate.

'Do you want a word with her?' I ask.

'Will she even remember what I say? Nah, I won't bother.'

I envy my sister her ability to pack my mother into such a pragmatic, practical space as this, Mam not even worth a few moments of chat. 'OK,' I say, 'all right.' But I'm disappointed in Imy, in her lack of care for our mother. For me.

As time goes on, Mam forgets to change from her nightdress into clothes, so I start to visit daily to pull her into trousers and jumpers. She forgets to bathe, too, so I manoeuvre her into the bath and wash her.

'I'm like a baby,' she says, poking at suds and smiling benignly, while I gently sponge her skin.

And, despite my ministrations, when I arrive at Mam's door each day, she is always surprised to see me.

'Oh, Sharon,' she says today, as if I haven't been in the longest time. 'Is Imy with you?'

'Nope,' I say, 'she's still living in Spain, Mam. In Bilbao.'

'Huh, Spain. Imagine. *Viva España*.'

I giggle. '*Viva España* for sure, Mam.'

'I've never liked travelling myself. All that running about,' she says, 'it'd exhaust you.'

'Is that right?'

I have learned not to contradict her. She often says things like this with absolute certainty though, sometimes, her pronouncements arrive with a doubtful, far-off look, as if she's trying to net the veracity of her words, but failing to catch anything. Other times, disconnected comments emerge, particles plucked from the silt of memories.

'Your father had womanly hands,' she says now, her tone dreamy, as she stares out the window.

I'm emptying the bin and I stand with the bag noosed in my hand, gripping it tighter. I say, airily, 'So, what was he like, this father of mine?' But she's already gone, ascended back into the cloud-place she occupies most of the time.

I see a fresh note taped to the press, to add to my more mundane ones for identifying appliance plugs and the contents of drawers:

'DO NOT FEED CAT. NOT MY CAT. (KILLS BIRDS).'

I smile, impressed by her lucidity, her directness. I turn to look at her trailing one finger across the windowpane, following the birds' movements from bath to feeder to fence. There is awe and joy in her face, and it strikes me she is becalmed, no more the rushing hawk of her younger years. Stillness suits her, makes her cheerier, a thing none of us would ever have believed.

'It'd be lovely to be able to fly, wouldn't it?' Mam says, lifting her face to me and smiling. She raises her arms like wings. 'Freedom!' she says, laughing.

*

I let myself into our flat above the Ennis butcher. I'm soaked from my run through the thunder shower, and I can hear Imy and Mam arguing. I'd like to get to the bedroom without them seeing me; I want to think more about what Emer has said about chaotic women. I push the living-room door softly, but Mam spots me.

'You're not taking us out of here,' Imy is saying. 'I'll refuse to go. Sharon will too.'

'We'll see about that,' Mam says.

'Yeah, we will. I'll see to it,' Imy barks.

'Do that so.'

Their familiar sparring wearies me.

'I'll get the authorities involved,' Imy says. 'Sister Paschal at the convent. All the nuns.'

'You'll do no such thing,' Mam says quietly, and her calm makes Imy boil.

'The inspector will stop you,' my sister shouts. 'It's illegal to be pulling children in and out of a million schools.'

Mam tuts and crosses her arms, as if waiting for Imy to say something useful.

'Is it true, Mam?' I ask, though I already know. 'Are we moving again?'

'Say goodbye to Beaky and her feathered friends,' Imy snaps.

'Her name's Emer,' I say.

'Who gives a shite, Sharon? It's over, we're gone. Mad Meg has decided County Clare's not for her.' She flicks her hand at Mam. 'Where to now, Amelia Earhart? What's the next great adventure?'

'Mam, do we have to leave? Really?' I ask. My gut starts up its ritual churn; I suck the ends of my hair. My mother has her determination face on, and I know we'll be in the car as soon as everything is packed. I flump onto the sofa. 'Why?' I say, unable to keep the whinge out of my voice. 'Why do you have to upend us, just when things are settling?'

Mam's hands flail and her face pinks. 'You girls see me as a carnival duck that you can shoot at.' The lisp has started, a sure sign of fury. 'A duck that'll just bob along, a smile on its face, despite your bullets.'

'Bullets?' shouts Imy. 'What are you on about, Mam? Who's shooting ducks? You're fucking mad!'

'Is it any wonder if I am mad?' Mam roars. 'You fire complaints at me constantly, Imy. You too, Sharon. I never met such critical girls.'

Imy snorts. 'We've reason to be. You never listen to what we want, you've no respect for us.' She goes up to Mam and pokes her chest. 'You don't give a fuck about anyone but yourself. You couldn't care less about me and Sharon.'

Mam slaps Imy's cheek so hard that I jump. 'And what about what *I* want, Imy?' she screams. 'What about me?' Tears bubble from her eyes. 'Who cares about *me*?'

*

I go to walk the prom in Salthill, as I do every morning, and the Atlantic – solid and wild beside me – is a comfort, as always. I look over the sea to Black Head and County Clare, breathe deep on the saline wind, and up my pace. I can see one other person ahead, a small figure with streeling hair, coming towards me. It takes me a few seconds to realise that I'm looking at my mother, out on this April morning, coat-less and bare-legged, miles from her flat, all a-trot as if abroad on important business.

I dash to her, calling out, 'Mam, Mam, what on earth? Where are you going? God almighty.' I pull off my jacket and go to push her arms through the sleeves. She holds up her fists for me to see the shells and gull feathers she's clutching.

'I'm going to decorate my kitchen,' she says.

'Oh, Mam.' I throw my jacket around her shoulders and lead her to where I've parked. Her feet slip-slap along the footpath and her legs are grey from cold. 'Bloody slippers,' I mutter.

Mam stops walking, stoops forward to look at her feet, then lifts her eyes to mine. 'I'm going spare, amn't I, Sharon?'

*

We go to Clones, County Monaghan. Every few years Mam brings us here and snails through the place, looking intently at every building, exploring each street. We crawl the town and Mam surveys in silence; we never get out of the car, and we don't visit anyone. Imy used to ask if any of our relatives were in Clones, but Mam wouldn't say and, today, Imy is too sulky to bother. I read the names on the shopfronts and pubs, and wonder if any of these McQuillans, Earls, or Hamiltons are our people and, if they are, whether they ever think of us.

Today Mam takes a hill in the town and turns into the grounds of a church. She drives the car right to where the cemetery begins and gets out.

'Stay here, girls.'

I watch her flit from plot to plot, crouching in front of gravestones to read their inscriptions.

'It's as if she's looking for a specific grave,' I say.

'The cadaver hunter,' Imy says, putting on her Walkman headphones and slumping low in the seat.

I get out of the car and follow Mam from a distance, watching her dodge behind Celtic crosses and crestfallen angels, wings cocked, arms outspread. I try to imagine a young Mam here, a girl a bit like me, wandery, chatting with herself, the way I do, her head lax and cottony. I get distracted by sunny lichen blossoms on headstones and by the pippity song of a blackbird.

'Saffron beak,' I say. 'Glossy black plumage.'

'*It's-me-it's-me-it's-me,*' the blackbird replies.

I glance at Mam up ahead of me, as if through mist, and I'm astonished to see that her arms are around another person, a woman. I come up closer. Mam is hugging this woman hard, whoever she is, and they are rocking in each other's arms, and laughing noisily. Mam doesn't laugh like this, and she doesn't have friends. Other women are to be avoided. I step out onto the path to make myself known, but they don't see me, and then Mam and the woman are fully kissing, the way soap stars kiss, eyes closed, hungry tongues clashing. I stagger backwards, but I'm mesmerised by the crush of their mouths, and I can't look away. I've never known Mam to embrace anyone but Imy and me. She's off-guard, loose, wild as a bird. She is kissing this woman like a lover and, though my shock is absolute, I find I don't disapprove because, for once, Mam looks lost and happy, instead of just lost. The woman ends their kiss and, holding Mam by the shoulders, she looks deep into her face.

'Meggy,' she says, rivers flowing down her cheeks, and Mam is crying too, real, streaming tears. 'Oh, Meg.'

And they laugh again, school-girlish titters, and they hug and sway, and then the woman sees me, and she stops all movement. Mam turns her head, spies me, and scowls. She pulls herself out of the woman's arms and marches towards me.

'That's your father,' she hisses, flinging her hand at a cross-shadowed grave. 'Imy's too.' She stalks back the way we came, and I stare at the well-kept grave, evenly planted with begonias along its sides. I look up and the woman is gone. I step around the cross to read the name.

*

'Tell me about the Clones doctor, Mam,' I say.

She has just asked me yet again if she can get me something to eat. She has been changing the TV channel every few minutes, and I want to divert her.

'Clones?'

'The doctor there. In the graveyard. You told me he was my father. And Imy's.'

'Is that a place – Clones?'

I sigh. 'Yes, in Monaghan, remember?'

'Wait now.' She frowns. 'Monaghan. And was I there once?'

*

Imy and I can't agree on what to do with the ashes.

'Can you not just stick her on your mantelpiece?' Imy glances to my fireplace. 'Where is she now?'

'In my wardrobe.'

'Ooh, bold Sharon. Meg would do her nut.' Imy looks ceiling-ward, then changes her mind and addresses the floor. 'You'd hate that, wouldn't you, Meg, being all quiet and ignored in some dark corner?'

'I don't want Mam stuck on the mantelpiece, like a useless gew-gaw.'

'She'd hardly be that.' Imy rolls her eyes. 'Let's just decide now. Come on.'

I go to the sideboard and bring two small wooden boxes I've bought to the sofa. 'Why don't we divide her equally between these? I'll keep one box and you take the other back to Bilbao.'

'Split her in half?' Imy shakes her head. 'Is that a bit weird?'

'Maybe.' I think again. 'We could bring her where she was happiest, then. Scatter her.'

'Was Meg ever happy, though?'

'Ah Imy, help me. I'm trying.'

My sister grimaces. 'Well, which places did she like, Sharon? You tell me. I haven't a clue.'

'Monaghan? Or County Clare, maybe? We all liked Ennis.'

Imy stands up and grabs her jacket. 'Listen, I don't give a shite what you do. Let her stay in the wardrobe. Seriously. She's no use to me.'

*

Today Mam is trying to remember where she comes from. 'It's up the way,' she says, pointing to the ceiling.

'Heaven?' I tease. 'The air? Or did you come down from a nest, Mam? A bird baby.'

'No, Sharon, up, up. On the map.'

'Monaghan,' I say.

'Yes, that's it. Monaghan.' She closes her eyes and smiles. 'And, before that, Maumakeogh.'

I look at her. 'Maumakeogh? Really? First mention of that, Mam.'

'Oh yes. Maumakeogh. The misty pass.'

'And where's that?' I ask.

'In Mayo. There, above the sea.'

I peer at her closed eyes and the beatific set to her mouth. She looks placid, content. All this memory-loosening may have brought an ease to her; an ability to rest, to stop running from the shadows that have always crowded in her wake. But I know I'm losing her, too. She's fading. And I know that because she is more reduced, less able for the smaller things like dressing and using the toilet, soon Imy and I will have to make the decision to put her somewhere; choose her final home.

Every day I come to Mam's flat to help and to sit with her, and every time she's quieter, further retreated, than the last. She is busily exiting into some place where no one can follow. And I want, with all my heart, to reach a rope down and pull her back up. Just for a while. I want to winkle from her all of the things that she concealed, and I never tried to uncover. I want, mostly, to ask my mother who she is. Who

I am. Where we fit in. But it's too late, I know. I didn't insist on those revelations soon enough, and Mam's descent into a completely private elsewhere, some halcyon place, is now too long underway.

The bird book lies open on her lap. 'What are you looking at?' I ask. 'Which bird?'

Mam's eyes don't open; she has drifted into one of her unbidden naps, and I want to leave her there, in the cushion of sleep. I pick up the book and examine the page.

Alcedo atthis. Kingfisher.

*

A Madeira-wine sunset, golden and warm, lights up Liscannor Bay. We took the love-knotted roads of the Burren to get here, Imy driving and me holding the urn. We sang 'She'll be comin' 'round the mountain' and I held up the urn to sway it along to the beat, until Imy and I nearly choked on our giggles and snorts.

Imy stops the car above the sea and points to where the cliffs run out. 'Hag's Head,' she says. 'Appropriate.'

Annoyance whips my heart. 'You don't always have to make something bad of Mam, Imy. You could be nicer.'

'I know I could, Sharon,' she says, 'but what am I supposed to do? All our lives Meg disrupted us, pulled us back and forth, took out her disappointments on us. You said yourself you blame her. She was a crap mother; nothing changes that.'

'She had her moments,' I say, casting around for good. 'She was gentler towards the end, you know, softer. Mostly. And she loved us. We know that much.'

Imy sighs. 'Well, maybe she did and maybe she didn't. What exactly is love?'

I glance at my sister. 'Imy, remember that time we went to the graveyard in Clones, after the great Ennis escape?'

'Yeah.'

'Mam told me something.'

'Did she now?' Imy stares out over the Atlantic, beating its way to the shore. 'What did she tell you?'

'She said who our father was.' Imy's hard-knuckle grip on the steering wheel is just like Mam's, the same stressed-out clamp. She puts her forehead to the wheel.

'Well?' she says.

I look out at the heaving sea. 'A married doctor in Clones. Years older than her. Long dead.'

Imy parps a breath through her lips. 'So that's that.'

'She also told me she came from Mayo originally.'

'Jesus fuck, we really knew nothing about her.'

'Nothing. And never will now.'

Imy looks at me and grabs my hand. 'Come on.'

We get out of the car and walk the rough cliff path, the wind lifting our hair. I hold the urn tight to my chest and tuck my free arm through Imy's.

'They say kingfishers foretell death,' I tell her. 'And they become even more beautiful when they die. Their plumage renews itself, gets plumper, glossier.' My sister grunts. 'Imagine, Imy, all that russet and sapphire.'

'Do you think Mam's out there somewhere, Sharon, putting on new feathers?'

'Maybe.'

Imy laughs. 'Knowing Meg, she most likely is.'

We kneel at the top of the cliff and Imy opens the urn lid with the car key. She puts her two hands over mine, on the pot. I nod and my sister nods too. We hoosh the ashes to the waiting water and, as we do, the sunset flares to a deep orange.

'Goodbye, Mam,' I call.

'Safe travels, Meg,' Imy says.

And out she goes, our beautiful mother, out over the sea and into the sun, glorious as any kingfisher, diving into the blue.

Downbeat

Chris Wright

Niamh turned the Merc onto the motorway. She loved the motorway. The sheer concrete monotony of it. She could hear the samba in it – 2/4 time to 100 beats per minute – with the soft intro a slow rumble as the ground changed beneath the tyres. The way it sped and slowed with traffic. The waltz of lanes, the sway of notes, the emotion between drivers encroaching upon one another. It was beautiful. Even the colour of concrete matched her trouser suit.

She was eleven years old again, getting ready for her first dance competition. She was so excited, practising in her bedroom every day, trying to pad her feet but losing control in the grasp of the music until she thumped too hard and Dad guldered up the stairs for her to cut it out. Mum surprised her with the perfect outfit – a Zeta ballroom skirt in pale turquoise twinkle with a custom crêpe leotard – and sat her on her knee, applying thick costume make-up with a trembling hand so she could look like the older girls. Niamh had never felt so beautiful. She even managed to ignore the prick of bone from her sick mother's knees, poking her in the back of the thigh.

They'd crept down the stairs, giggling, secretive fingers to mouths, Mum leaning against the wall at the bottom with raggedy breath, mouthing, go on, show Daddy. Niamh slipped into the living room. He was watching the news, mumbling words she didn't understand, like 'recession' and 'bailout,' and ones she did, like 'liar' and 'bastard' and 'ruined'. He took a long, crackling draw on his cigarette, a swig of liquid from a tall glass, swallowed and exhaled heavily. He didn't even turn his head.

She unconsciously wiped at her mouth with the back of her hand. A noise escaped, somewhere between a sigh and a grunt.

Too much? the man in the back said, stopping the speech he'd been practising, mid-sentence.

Hmmm?

Niamh regarded him in the rear-view, squinting her eyes and clenching her lips until they turned pale and thin like her fingernails. She shook her head. Her cradled phone buzzed and lit up with a message.

Can't make it 2 dads l8r. Could you call on way home? Thanks x

Anna, shirking her responsibilities again with a redundant question mark. Third time in as many weeks. No apology. No explanation. Typical Anna. Mum had always made excuses for her. She was too young to understand his anger. It was often left to Niamh to comfort her wailing sister.

Niamh ignored the message. She ran her thumb back and forth across a jag on the nail of her middle finger as the car slipped under the overpass. The glare of orange lights that lined the short tunnel slid in and out of the window like a photocopier.

The man in the back's phone cheeped. He answered it with a flourish.

Dan. Dan the man. Yes, Dan. Absolutely, Dan. I'm in the car. On my way to the office … just a few more days, Dan … uh-huh … uh-huh … what are you worried about, Dan? Sure, you pay less tax than Bezos, ha ha ha.

Niamh kept her eyes on the road ahead as it curved to the right, the docks springing into view: sharp, industrial buildings, shimmering in the piss yellow hue of the winter sun.

It wasn't long before his phone rang again.

Sean, big Sean, sure as Sean. Aye … aye … yeah, the only thing I'll be redistributing will be my shares … ha ha ha. Yeah … yup … of course. I'll see you soon … Sean … bye Sean, bye bye bye bye.

The man lifted a newspaper from the pile beside him, his face red as he tried to stifle a grin. Man of the people, indeed, he said holding up the front page, the picture of him almost identical to his real face in the back seat, the smile well honed.

Not long now. The big day. The vote to end all votes. I can get you into the chamber, you know. See how it all works. Democracy in action.

Politics? Sure, it's Peking Opera to me, she said.

But this changes everything. They're clambering to get in to witness it.

She shook her head and grimaced.

It's history, he said.

A message pinged onto her phone screen.

What time will you be home later?

It's two cats fighting in an alley, Niamh said.

I wouldn't expect someone like you to get it, he replied, before snapping open the newspaper. They drove the rest of the way in silence.

***

After work she weaved through the labyrinthine estate at the city's periphery – waltz, 3/4 time to 84–90 beats per minute – until she arrived at the block of flats, right at the centre. She walked quickly from the car to the flat and hesitated as she lifted her fist to rap the door, trying the handle instead. It opened.

Dad? she called, her body tingling with the usual nervous energy. She was sure that she'd find him cold someday soon. Dad, she called again.

A splutter and cough echoed down the hall.

Jesus, Dad, she said, entering the living room. He didn't even turn. She opened the windows to let out the hot smell. Then she asked him the questions he once asked her.

Have you washed today?

Have you cleaned your teeth?

Have you eaten?

Why not?

Leave me be, he said, waving a hand as if accosted by a fly, before returning his hazy stare to the TV.

Where's yer ma? he asked, the words straining his vocal cords.

There was a time when Niamh would've sat him down and broken the news to him every day as if it had just happened. Now she flung the words at him, She's dead, Dad, and let him sort himself out. The distraction gave her a chance to put away the meal replacement shakes she'd bought at the Tesco Express down the road. She opened the fridge door and recoiled.

You need to remember to throw out the old milk, she shouted, but he wasn't listening. His grief had drained away as quickly as it came; the sudden change signalled by the flick of a lighter and the crackle of burning tobacco.

And you shouldn't be smoking, she said as she came back into the room with a milkshake.

Where's yer sister?

She couldn't make it.

Why not?

She didn't say.

Off whorin' with that fella again.

Dad, please. I haven't got time for this.

Niamh checked her phone. A message from Brian. She hadn't even heard it ding.

I thought you were coming straight home after work. Can you let me know what time you'll be in?

She replied, *Soon*, and put her phone back in her pocket.

I have to go, Dad. Don't you want to see the car?

What car?

The Merc. You love the Merc.

His eyes glazed and he sniffed the air like it had changed around him.

I had a Merc once. God, I loved that car.

I know, Dad, she said, but he didn't hear.

It's how I met my wife, Deirdre.

Yes, Mum, I know.

Near hit her with it. Screeched to a halt in front of her. Told her she had a face that could stop traffic. She laughed and asked me if that was a compliment or not. Of course, it was a compliment. She was a stunner. I dropped her home, her auld bastard of a da glarin' at me as she went inside. He always hated me, he said with a rueful smirk. Called me Flash.

I know, Dad. I remember.

I showed him. Sold so many I was able to buy it outright.

He took a long draw of his cigarette.

Okay, Dad. Drink your shake. It's strawberry. Your favourite.

He looked at her, confused, then at the shake. His face changed. I'm not fallin' fer that, he said, dropping his cigarette in the shake with a plop and a fizz and grinning at her through broken grate teeth.

Fuck's sake, Dad.

***

Niamh slipped into the house, expecting the usual rumble – the girls fighting over whose turn it was with the iPad, Brian shouting at them, them not paying any notice – but she was met with an imposing silence.

There you are, Brian said in a cooing voice, sticking his head around the kitchen door.

What's this? she asked.

His face straightened as he stepped out from behind the door.

What d'you mean? I've made dinner.

I thought we were ordering in.

Jesus Christ, Niamh, I was trying to do something nice.

Sorry, sorry. One of those days, she said, painting on a smile. Anna couldn't sort Dad, so I had to do it.

Again?

Yes, again. And he still thinks I'm trying to poison him.

Isn't it about time you got him some proper help?

Can we just … not?

They ate dinner – his speciality, he called it. Carbonara with a cheap Pinot Grigio, a Rolo and a weak coffee after – in near silence. It was only when the quiet burned extra hot that they exchanged information about their day with stories as bland as the pasta. Niamh twirled thick spaghetti around her fork while he talked, slopping it off the end. She repeated the process several times before committing to a mouthful.

Brian pulled a newspaper from his bag and dropped it onto the table.

I saw this at the office. Had to laugh.

He paused for her to get a good look at the front page she'd already seen.

Man of the people, my hole, he continued.

I only drive him.

Didn't the Nazis say that? I was only driving Hitler to work, honest.

He said the last part in a silly voice. He sometimes did that, cut her to the bone.

Do you want me to quit? she asked.

I don't *want* you to do anything, but I think you want to. Being around that man. It's making you miserable.

I'm fine.

He took her hand. His sympathetic touch made her jaw tighten. She pulled free.

We don't really need the money, he said.

Her stomach clenched. She glared at the bubbles riding on the oily surface of her black coffee.

Tell me this. If you could do anything, absolutely anything, what would it be? he asked.

Niamh threw her coffee down the sink and left the room.

***

Niamh and Brian sat in front of the TV, each perched on their own sofa; him watching intently, her barely seeing anything past her phone. Every so often he would turn to explain something that didn't need explaining. He'd catch her face lit up in the glow from her phone screen and sigh loudly until she slipped it between her leg and the arm rest. She'd wave her hands like a retiring blackjack dealer and feign interest in whatever nonsense was on the screen.

They went to bed. He initiated sex. She went along with it because she couldn't deal with the look on his face when she refused again. They went through the usual repertoire. Wet kisses, mistaking pain for passion. Hard grabbing and tugging. Rough fingers too quick into her. She retreated, distracting him by taking the head of his penis into her mouth and rolling it around for a few minutes. He feigned ecstatic moans of encouragement. No sooner had she taken it from her lips than he was on top, thrusting hard into her – rumba, 4/4 time to

92–100 beats per minute – her grimace lost in the dark of the room. The judder and twitch came fast, and he collapsed on top of her. She was thankful he was quick. One last peck on the side of the mouth and he was away to the bathroom to clean himself off. Then he went back downstairs for a couple more hours of TV while she navigated a fractured sleep.

***

Niamh awoke and slipped a hand across to his side of the bed only to find it cold. She drifted in and out of sleep for another fifteen minutes before dragging herself over to the window. The driveway was dark and wet, except for a light patch where Brian's van had sat overnight. She felt her chest loosen. He must have had an early call.

She went to the loo, sitting for longer than necessary while she checked her social media. Her phone gave an enthusiastic trill as a message from Janey appeared on the screen.

You still on 4 coffee?

Niamh had forgotten they'd made plans. She considered putting Janey off. She'd rather spend the day in her pyjamas, bingeing her favourite show on Netflix while not actually watching, instead browsing shopping sites, filling baskets only to delete them. Then again, she had been craving company of late.

***

Niamh entered the coffee shop twenty minutes late which, for her, was practically early. Janey sat at a table near the back, face in a novel, front cover curled around and clamped tight in one hand, a small coffee in the other. She was wearing her usual sports gear. Black leggings, purple T-shirt and black gilet fleece that had never seen the inside of a gym. Her hair was pulled back in a tight ponytail. She looked up and waved enthusiastically.

Hey babe, she said, standing to squeeze Niamh in a tight hug. Haven't seen you in ages. You look good.

I look terrible. You've lost weight.

Thanks. A few pounds.

No more, now. You don't want people thinking you're ill.

Janey sat down, a little bit of the bounce taken out of her, while Niamh ordered a coffee, black.

So, what's the biz, fizzy Liz? Janey asked.

Not much.

Ach, come on. There must be something.

Honestly, very little.

How's work?

Niamh rolled her eyes and swallowed, hoping to bury the threat of tears.

That bad, huh? Funny, I thought about you the other day when I saw yer man on the news. I says to Simon, I says, Must be wile interesting drivin' him around like Niamh does. Especially with this vote they're all talking about.

What did Simon say?

Who's he? What vote? Where am I?

They both laughed.

The joys of the younger man, Janey said, cradling her cup between both hands.

The waitress set a coffee down in front of Niamh. It sloshed from side to side, splashing over the rim and onto the saucer. Niamh shook her head, the waitress none the wiser.

It's not half as exciting as you'd think, driving him around. I doubt he even remembers my name.

How long have you been driving him for?

Him, eh? Niamh tallied in her head. Eighteen months.

What's he like, you know, behind the scenes? Janey asked, putting her cup to her lips, and widening her eyes.

He's … he's a typical politician. Needs a good dose of reality if you ask me.

Tell me this. Would you vote for him?

No, Niamh replied.

Janey took a long sip of coffee, allowing Niamh the option of giving more detail but silence filled the space between them.

You still on for dance class tomorrow night? Janey asked.

Niamh shook her head.

Ach, come on. You haven't been in ages. They were your idea.

I can't make it.

But it's the *paso doble*. To *España Cañi*. You were looking forward to this one, Janey said, clicking her fingers above her head and grinning.

Niamh fought a smile. We'll see, she replied. So, what's new with you?

Janey droned on about her post-divorce love life and her job. Niamh found her concentration waning. The noise of the coffee shop swelled around her until it engulfed Janey's words. Mumbled conversations, rattling dishes, an unsettled child, the waitress's clicky shoes all dragged together into a rhythm she counted in her head – quickstep, 4/4 time to 192–208 beats per minute – her leg trembling and her feet burning with the urge to move. She gulped down half her tepid coffee and did her best to concentrate on the conversation.

… sure, as Kondo says, if it doesn't bring you joy, buck it out …

Who?

Yer woman off the telly. She says if something doesn't spark joy, get rid of it. Although she also says you should have no more than thirty books. I mean, seriously? Thirty in each room, maybe. She laughed long and hard at her own joke. Niamh managed a subdued smile.

You should buck yer man out, Janey said.

Aye, of the car.

They both chuckled.

When Dave was in AA, before the divorce, he used to repeat this mantra thingy. What was it again?

Janey's eyes roamed the room as she searched for the words.

He had it up on the wall. It was something like, Give us the serenity to accept the things we cannot change, courage to change the things we can, and wisdom to know the difference. Little did he know he was giving me ideas.

Janey sipped. I took back control alright, she said. Maybe it's time you did too. You always did love a good key change.

Niamh laughed. She opened her mouth to follow up with a joke of her own but was interrupted by her phone, buzzing on the table. She tilted it to take a quick look.

WTF Niamh? Dad says you swore at him and left. He was really upset. And can you stop giving him those milkshakes? They're full of sugar.

She held up the message for Janey to read.

Janey made a non-committal noise.

Sure, she's the one who brings him cigarettes so he can smoke his brains out but thinks a bit of lettuce will fix him, Niamh said, still staring at her phone.

Janey downed the dregs of her coffee and checked her watch.

***

Niamh pulled up in front of the hotel. Her boss stayed there on workdays at the taxpayers' expense. She messaged to let him know she was outside. A few minutes later he bumbled out the door, phone at his ear, a newspaper over his head to protect him from the rain. His nasal voice cut right through her and the closed window.

Bill, Billy boy. It's in the bag, Bill. Start the paperwork. We'll be sorted come the morning … aye … ha … you can buy two.

When Niamh had first started driving for him, she'd get out and open the door. A few days in and she was told not to do it anymore. They didn't want pictures in the paper of a woman opening the door for him.

He ran to the car and reached for the door handle.

Click.

She looked down, surprised to see her own finger on the central locking button.

He yanked the handle again, hard. And again. And again.

She was frozen to the seat, adrenaline building in her belly.

It's locked, he shouted.

She didn't even look round.

Hello? Eh … Miss?

She gritted her teeth, unsure how many times she had told him her name.

I've a press call in an hour. Can you open the door, please?

The same rogue finger that locked the doors started the engine.

Jesus Christ, I'm getting soaked, he said, reverting to the accent he tried to hide. He rattled hard at the handle. I'm serious, young lady. Open the door or you'll never work in this industry again. I know people, the man shouted through the window, his face twisted and red.

Niamh pressed the voice command button on the steering wheel.

'Play *España Cañi*,' she said.

The music started, drowning out his threats and filling the car with sweet, familiar notes. Niamh took a deep breath and let the sound of the Spanish Gypsy Dance fill her bones with a warmth she hadn't felt in years. She lifted a small bag from the door pocket, took out an old lipstick from the bottom and applied it carefully. She smacked her lips together and flicked on the indicator, glancing over her shoulder, and pulling into a gap in the thickening morning traffic.

***

Niamh arrived at her dad's flat and stepped out of the car into the thumping rain, two stacked coffees balanced precariously in one hand and two sausage baps in polystyrene burger boxes in the other.

Dad was fast asleep on the sofa. His bony hand sat curled on top of his chest, rising and falling with the sway of his shallow breath. Thick skin bunched and hung at the knuckles, his flesh spotted, pitted and lined in blue veins like a confluence on a map.

She barely recognised this half-man, curled up on the chair. He looked like a dead bird in the road.

He awoke with a cough when she flicked off the TV.

… was watching 'at.

He recoiled when she turned on the big light.

I've brought you breakfast, she said, setting the boxes down in front of him.

Wha' for? he said, wiping his chin with the back of a hand.

I know what Anna's been trying to feed you.

Thon rabbit food, he mumbled.

She popped the top off the box, revealing a packed sausage bap. She handed it to him. He didn't hesitate. Oily fat mixed with brown sauce and ran down his chin on the first bite.

'Member when we ate those big baps yer ma packed for us when we were at Levante beach? he said.

Yes, Dad. Sure didn't Anna drop hers in the sand? She cried her eyes out.

Niamh pulled a tissue from her pocket and wiped the sauce from his chin.

You gave her yours, didn't you? he said.

Niamh smiled and nodded, offering up the silence for him to paddle in the warmth of his memories. She stared at the TV instead, a smile gathering at clips from the latest celebrity dance show.

Dad clicked his fingers and pointed at the screen.

I love this show.

Niamh looked at him.

Really? The dancing show. You watch that?

Yeah, takes me right back. My daughter, Niamh, she was a wonderful dancer when she was wee. Made me so proud. She looked just like her mother, before she got sick that is. After that it was hard …

He stopped. His lip quivered. Niamh spotted something familiar in the look on his face. Her girls. A skinned knee or a bad word from a boy in school bringing out the same pained expression. She turned back to the TV to hide her own tears.

She took her phone from her pocket and typed out a message to Janey.

See you in class x

Niamh hit send. She returned her phone to her pocket, wiped her face, and stood.

Right you, let's get you dressed, she said, holding out her hand.

Where we going?

I'm taking you out in the Merc. We can drive slowly past Grandpa's house if you want.

He smiled and took her hand.

Niamh helped him up from the sofa, placing her free hand on his side for balance.

I had a Merc once, he said. God, I loved that car. It's how I met my wife, Deirdre …

People Who Want History Want *History*

Naomi Krüger

Beechwood House Dementia Care Home

Reminiscence Interview with Edward P
Conducted by: Justyna C

[Recording started at 11:04]

J: [Inaudible]

E: … You never buy a door to fit a space, you always make
the space to fit the door. That's if you want the door to
hang properly. Maybe they don't. Who knows with these
people? These couples coming in together, all wide-eyed
and matchy-matchy. Looking for an old door for their new
downstairs bog or the bedroom in the extension, looking
for a door with character. And they'd hand over some
bullshit calculations on a scrap of paper. I'd look at them
and shake my head and say, sorry mate, no can do. We don't
have any doors for those measurements. You should've seen
their faces. [Laughs] They'd do this slow look around, gobs
wide open, taking them all in. Hundreds and hundreds.

Lined up, one after the next and the next. Porch doors with coloured glass, nice six-panelled jobs with proper mouldings. Victorian, Edwardian. The ones pretending to be older. Cottagey ledge-and-brace numbers made out of solid oak. All too good for the likes of them. Water, water everywhere and not a drop to drink. [Laughs] … Are you getting all this down, love?

J: I'm sorry. I'll be with you …. [cups clinking] I'm just bringing the tea.

E: Tea? You want me to spill my guts, give you these nuggets of wisdom, and tea's the best you can do?

J: We have juice if you prefer. And biscuits.

E: I'm not being funny, love – what's your name again?

J: Justyna.

E: I'm not being funny Jus-teen-ah, but I would like to submit a formal request for something a teensy bit stronger.

J: I don't think we … I don't think I can help you with that. My colleague … the other lady … will be in soon. I'm only keeping things … I'm only waiting–

E: Like that, is it? Waiting for the big boss? I'll have to be careful, then. Have to mind my Ps and Qs. Last time I was in a room like this I was on my best behaviour. No comment officer, no comment, no comment, no comment. [Laughs]

J: Oh – I'm not a police officer. You're not in any trouble.

E: I realise that, love. I worked that out all by myself.

J: [Inaudible]

E: Can't picture you wrestling anyone to the ground … and that thing in your nose would be ripped out in no time.

[Door opens. Inaudible voices]

E: Who's that? What's going on now then?

J: That was Denise. She's been held up. She said we should get started without her.

E: The sooner we start, the sooner we ...

J: Let me just gather ... [inaudible] I'm just here to find out ... just here to ask you some questions about your life.

E: Jesus. Which bits?

J: Well ... er. Why don't you tell me? ... Why don't we start with your family?

E: My family? My *Family*? There was no family. There was only me and Burt. My brother. Older by seven years and didn't he just milk it? What d'you want to know about him for? We never got on. He never really gave me any credit. All it takes, sometimes, is one mistake. One fucking mistake, and that's it. People know you as the lad who lit his cigarette too close to the varnishes for the rest of your fucking life. [Fist banging on table]

J: Alright. Okay. We can talk about something else. Tell me more about your work, maybe?

E: You want me to tell you about my work?

J: Yes. Please. I'd like to hear it.

E: Would you? Planning to go into joinery are you? Is that why you're taking notes?

J: No ... I just want to hear about ... your experiences, the things you remember.

E: The things I remember.

J: I thought you might enjoy sharing–

E: I'll make you a deal. A story for a story. I tell you one thing, and you tell me something in return.

J: That's not what we're supposed to be doing–

E: Who says?

J: Denise – there's a framework for this and we only have half an hour. I–

E: Alright then, Jeanie, if you insist. Ask and ye shall receive. Knock, and it shall be opened unto you. [Sound of knocking on the table]

J: Sorry? I don't–

E: Come on, keep up! I say 'knock, knock', you say, 'who's there?'

J: Ah, okay. A joke.

E: That's right. You're a fast learner. We'll try again, shall we? Knock, knock …

J: Who's there?

E: Nunya.

J: Nunya … who?

E: Nunya fucking business. [Laughs]

J: [Inaudible]

E: [Still laughing] Ah, come on, Julie. Don't be like that. Don't take it so personally … I'm only messing with you. A man can't say anything these days. I swear–

J: I think we should have a little break. Only a little one. I think it's better. I'll just turn this off for a min–

[Recording stopped at 11:15]

Beechwood House Staff Manual p. 68

Tips for Conducting Reminiscence Interviews with New Residents:

1. Although people with dementia typically find it easier to recall long-term rather than short-term memories, they may still find direct questions stressful. Instead of asking 'Do you remember your first job?' for example, you might instead share a short story about a job you've had and how it felt to learn new skills. This may give the

resident time to pick up 'conversational cues' in a more natural way.

2.   Some useful topics to begin your interview include: working life, home life, sport and other social activities, home town, living conditions and memories of significant places. Topics to approach with caution include religion, politics and specific family members (unless first mentioned by the resident themselves).

3.   Occasionally, a resident may recall a painful or traumatic memory or stray into uncomfortable territory. Although it is important to listen, if a resident becomes distressed or fixated on inappropriate memories, you are strongly encouraged to change the topic or find another way to distract them so you can return to more neutral ground.

4.   Remember that sometimes words are not enough. Photographs and other items can be excellent triggers for memory. You might also use music or encourage a resident to 'act out' a familiar routine or work practice.

5.   Don't forget to press record!

[Recording restarted at 11:21]

E: ... I have my tea, I have my biscuit. I'm on my best behaviour and ready to do your bidding.

J: I just want to ask you some questions.

E: And I, as your obedient servant will be happy to ... comply.

J: Okay. Let's start with work then. Can you tell me about what it was like when you first started? ... Like, for instance, when I first started university, I worked in a restaurant for a bit. Not a restaurant, really, just a café. I did barista training – that's when you learn to make the coffee and what order to do it in and you have to make sure the fridge is always stocked, and the pots don't get too backed up, and you have to remember all the orders as they come in. And I think I did get better over time. My manager said I was starting to use my own initiative – but then they just stopped giving me hours. They stopped putting me on the rota, so now I work here–

E: Did you say university?

J: Yes.

E: A clever one, eh? I've always liked the clever ones. Women with a spark in their eyes.

J: I'm studying English.

E: Your English sounds fine to me, love.

J: It is. I mean, I've been here since I was young. I'm studying literature.

E: Lit-er-a-ture, eh?

J: Yes.

E: Books and whatnot. Tell me a story, then.

J: No – not like that. I don't write them.

E: But you read them, don't you?

J: Yes, but I don't … I'm here to hear *your* stories.

E: An eye for an eye, a tooth for a tooth.

J: Sorry?

E: Give a little, take a little.

J: You want me to tell you a story?

E: You catch on quick.

J: We don't have time.

E: Ladies first. A story for a story.

J: Okay. Well. I've been re-reading some Polish folk tales recently. Ones my parents used to tell me. It's for an assignment at uni. The way traditional stories can change over time and how they can be read differently–

E: Chop, chop, Judy. Speed it up, will you.

J: Okay. Alright. So. There's this baker with three beautiful daughters: one who sings like a bird, one who makes the most delicious bread in the world, and one who tells stories

52

so good they enchant anyone who happens to hear them.

E: If only we had her here now, eh. [Laughs]

J: Should I stop?

E: No, no. Don't take on so easily. I'll zip my mouth, see. You go ahead. Don't mind me at all.

J: Well, soon enough an evil sorcerer sees the sisters over the garden fence and decides to trick them into marrying him one by one, so he can capture their souls and keep them locked up in his castle.

E: There's always one.

J: He disguises himself as a handsome prince. Or maybe it's a merchant. Either way, he looks rich enough that the father doesn't hesitate before offering the hand of the first daughter. The sorcerer rides away with her ... wait, no. I always leave out this bit. First, he casts a spell on her sisters and father, so they won't ... so that when he goes back for the others later they won't ... think anything of it–

E: Did you say you had any whiskey?

J: No. Only tea. Want some more?

E: [Inaudible]

J: Or another biscuit?

E: Nothing. You have nothing I want.

J: Right. I think that's enough from me, then. It's your turn now. Why don't you tell me about the place you used to work?

E: The family business?

J: Yes.

E: Are you sure?

J: What?

E: Are you sure you really want to know?

J: Yes, of course. Go ahead.

E: What you have to understand, Jeanie, is that the business wasn't always mine. And we didn't always specialise in doors. When we started out it was all sorts of things. Antiques and brass, furniture and fittings, fireplaces and coal buckets. My brother Burt had a friend who worked for a funeral place. Funeral Pete, I called him. Burt called him The Ferryman. He was always trying to be clever ...

J: So, you had an antique shop?

E: Nothing that grand. A workshop more like. *Pye and Sons, Restoration Specialists Since 1899.*

J: A family business.

E: Exactly. That's exactly what I was going for. Burt wasn't happy about it when I had the sign made. But I told him, I said, Burt – people who want history, want *history*. They want to believe we had our expertise passed to us through the blood. What does it matter if there's no father on the scene? What does it matter if we wouldn't piss on him if he was burning? It's the appearance that matters. And with Pete tipping us the wink every time he came across a juicy prospect, all those houses the council paid us to clear – we were getting by. More than getting by. On the up-and-up.

J: And the business kept growing?

E: We sold fittings and sundries, antiques and brass. I had a sign made. *Pye and Sons, Restoration Specialists Since 1899.* I fixed furniture and sold on the best pieces to dealers. Burt kept the books and went to the houses with Funeral Pete to check out new stock. We could've gone on like that forever if it wasn't for the fire.

J: The fire?

E: Didn't I just say that?

J: Yes, but, er ... you don't need to say any more. Not if it's upsetting.

E: Well of course it was upsetting. It was a fucking fire. We nearly lost the whole bloody workshop. And of course, it was my fault. Because I was always the careless one, easily distracted, fly-by-the-seat-of-my-pants, no good, no-hoper ... but, like I said to Burt, at the end of the day it wasn't me who left the lids off the varnish, left the tins scattered all over the shop so anyone could trip over them in the dark. I was tipsy, not bladdered like he made out. And can I tell you something ...

J: Justyna.

E: Jus-teen-ah. Yes. Can I tell you something I don't say to many people?

J: Yes.

E: My brother Burt was a miserable bastard. There was something not quite right about him. In the head. But he was good at showing his best face to the world. No one would've suspected a thing. Nice, gentle, quiet. A paragon of the community. Not when it came to me, though. Not when it came to forgiving my mistakes. Sometimes, it felt like he was rooting for me to fail just so he could enjoy the fallout. He docked my wages for years after, you know, even though I was supposed to be a partner. My name on the sign just as much as his. Treated me like a lackey, like a teenage dogsbody. Sweeping and carrying. Loading the truck, watching the shop, and never let near anything important. I never had a scrap of money for myself. Not a scrap. What'll that do to you? It's no wonder I'm always the one who ends up being questioned.

J: But this is just ... you're not in trouble now. This is just to learn some things about you.

E: You want to get to know me better?

J: Yes.

E: A pretty lass like you?

J: So you can settle in here.

E: Settle in ... here?

J: Not this room. This whole place. The home. Your new home.

E: Jesus. Are you sure I can't order myself a whiskey?

J: [Inaudible]

E: What was I saying? What was I saying?

J: Your brother, Burt.

E: Yes. I got even with him eventually.

J: Even?

E: I'm not saying I'm proud of it. But I'm not not saying that either. Bring a child up in the way he should go and when he is old, he shall not depart from it.

J: Sorry?

E: I left my wallet there one day. At the workshop. I had a woman on the go. I'd promised her a trip to the pictures, and I stopped by, nipped in to get it from the office. And then I heard a noise. A strange kind of squeaking. Like someone was working away at something over and over. Turns out I was right. [Laughs] ... Turns out I was bloody right.

J: I don't understand.

E: I thought there was someone breaking into the place. So, I went towards the sound. Through the back room, past the things we weren't ready to sell yet, out to an old shed that we were always meaning to knock down. I opened the door and there was Burt. And Funeral Pete. My brother and The Ferryman. Going at it. You know. Getting to know each other in the *biblical* sense. Tangled up in all sorts of horrible shapes. I can still see their faces. I can still see the look they gave me. Terrified, they were. Shamed and terrified.

J: Right. Okay ...

E: [Laughs]

J: Why don't we talk about something else? Like ... [paper rustling] the town you grew up in. It says here you grew up in Blackburn. What was Blackburn like when you were a child?

E: … And I thought bingo! This is my chance. Because it was still illegal then, you know. Two men together. I thought, this is my one chance to get ahead. To get him off my back once and for all.

J: Or … any meals you liked. Your favourite food. There was still rationing then, wasn't there? Do you remember queuing up—

E: … So I said wouldn't the police be interested in what the respectable businessman – the senior partner of *Pye and Sons, Restoration Specialists Since 1899* – got up to of a weekend? And wouldn't it be a shame if Mrs Funeral Pete caught wind of such a nasty rumour? Wasn't it already bad enough she had to live with a husband who spent more time with the dead than the living? Wouldn't this just finish her right off?

J: Shall I tell you the end of my story now?

E: … Sorry?

J: About the sorcerer who tried to imprison the souls of the three sisters.

E: [Inaudible]

J: And he was successful with the first two. But the final sister was too clever for him. He wanted her to tell him stories so he could write them down and capture her talent. But she'd mix them up deliberately, she'd get things wrong. 'Once there was a beautiful bird in a cage,' she'd say, 'and also, a long time ago there was a woodcutter who had three sons. Or maybe it was seven daughters. And he gave the daughters a songbird to keep in a cage. Or was it that they sang like birds and that's why all the most handsome men in the kingdom came from far and wide?'

E: Jesus. Slow down, love. Have a glass of water or something.

J: That's exactly what she wanted.

E: A glass of water?

J: No. Confusion. Distraction. So the sorcerer would turn away for a moment and she could rescue her sisters.

E: Are you ... alright? Do you need me to call someone for you? No? Well then. What was I saying? I was telling you about the doors.

J: Yes, but we can talk about something else if you want—

E: See, when you're dealing with proper doors – antique ones, nice six-panelled Victorian jobs with proper decorative mouldings – you don't just buy one and slot it in. You can't just add a bit here and shave off a bit there, as if symmetry means nothing. You have to have respect. You buy the door first and build the frame specially. Not the other way around. Not unless the space is already the right size.

J: Right.

E: Look at these ones here. All glass and plywood. If you dipped one of them in caustic solution, there'd be nothing left. I always liked that bit. The bit after they get lifted out. After you spray them with the pressure washer. Woosh, woosh! After you apply the acid. At first all you smell is the chemicals. But give it a minute and the wood comes through. Like it's been stripped back to the beginning. Every now and then a little whiff of the forest ...

J: Beautiful.

E: Are you writing that down?

J: Yes. It's almost like poetry.

E: I always had a way with words. Even Burt had to admit that. But it got me into trouble. Sometimes the best thing to say is nothing at all. No comment. No comment.

J: I'm sorry but we're almost out of time—

E: It was suspicious they said, the way he died.

J: [Inaudible]

E: And was there anyone I knew who might have wanted to cause him harm? And I almost said yes. I wanted to fucking kill him most days. But I never did. I never would. I wasn't capable of it. Not in the way they were thinking at least. I never meant for any of it to happen.

J: I'm sorry. It's just ... lunch will be ready soon. And Denise wants me to clear the room.

E: Denise? Denise? Who the fuck is Denise?

J: [Inaudible]

E: There were hundreds of doors. Hundreds and hundreds. And a drawer full of keys. But none of them worked because we stripped out the handles, the locks and hinges and sold them all separate. You could make more that way. All I'm saying is things could've been different if he hadn't always been so ...

J: I think there might be apple crumble today–

E: All I needed was someone to step up and give me a bit of care, a bit of guidance. You can't live without love, can you? It's too much for anyone ... sometimes, I used to think if I could just find the right key ... if I could just ... if I could just ... re-hinge it, line it up nice and tighten the screws ... then we could ... then he'd see that I was worth something. That I was capable of more ... that I wasn't the kind of person who would really say those things. Not really. Not to anyone who matters. No comment, no comment. All mouth and no trousers. That's me. All mouth. All. Fucking. Mouth.

J: I'm sorry, but I really have to stop this now. Maybe we can come back on another day. I'm really sorry. I'm just going to turn this off–

[Recording ended at 12:03]

***

On the Threshold of Knowledge: The Door as a Site of Possibility in Polish Folk Tales

ENG320 Assignment 2
Student No: 209374

The preface to Jan Brzezinzki's 1959 collection of Polish Folktales – *Tales from the Birch Forest* – is accompanied by a striking illustration. In a luxurious palace, a beautiful woman crouches next to an ornate, multi-panelled door. One hand is reaching for her pocket, ready to take out a giant key. Behind the door, taking up at least a third of the page, is darkness; a simple expanse of black ink. The woman is peering through the keyhole. The expression on her face can be interpreted either as fear, confusion or determination. She may be overcome by the realisation of her future fate, or alternatively, she may already be planning the best way to rescue her two unfortunate sisters who were lured into the darkness and imprisoned by the evil sorcerer, Rarog. In the foreground of the image, almost small enough to be ignored, is a book with its pages torn and scattered. It is unclear whether she has ripped the book herself or if it is simply a symbolic object. This ambiguity seems appropriate, considering the many different possible interpretations of this neglected folk tale.

In this essay I will examine Brzezinski's retelling of 'The Baker's Talented Daughters' (itself an Eastern European retelling of 'Bluebeard') to explore the ways it conforms or departs from previous versions. Is this yet another warning to women about the dangers of curiosity and disobedience? Or is this closer to the more progressive versions of 'Bluebeard' in which women scheme their way out of trouble using superior levels of intelligence? I will argue that this folk tale is unique in the interpretive gaps it leaves for readers.

Here, the heroine could easily be a trickster playing on her confusion to delay and distract her captor. Equally, she could be someone in a real place of unknowing, a person whose failure of memory (inflicted by the sorcerer so she will not speculate on her older sisters' whereabouts) proves to be a life-saving asset, even if it is used passively. As she says when asked to tell her new husband another story on their wedding night, 'I used to know so many. But they are only pieces, now. Let me try for you, husband. Spare me and let me try.' (Brzezinzki: 37)

***

Our Commitment to You: Every Person Matters

At Beechwood House we value every resident as a unique individual who deserves understanding and respect. We recognise that someone with dementia is more than their illness. Each resident has a rich history they may not be fully able to communicate. As their mental abilities decline, residents may feel particularly confused and vulnerable. They may struggle with ordinary tasks that once came easily to them. It is important that we take some time getting to know the person they once were as well as the person they are now. As part of this process, we commit to targeted memory work with every new resident.* Here at Beechwood House, we value the details and we put people at the centre. Sometimes it is the small things that help to remind us all that every person is valuable and every person matters.

*If you would like to attend the reminiscence session or obtain a copy of the interview recording you MUST indicate this on the request form attached to this booklet.

To guarantee that your request is honoured we MUST receive this no later than three days before the admission of a new resident.

***

Identity Plaque Proforma for New Residents
Completed by: Denise T

> **My name is:** Edward Pye
> **I prefer to be called:** Eddie
> **I like:** Talking about my old job. I used to repair antiques and I know a lot about restoring and fitting doors. In my past I was known as a 'Jack the Lad' and still like to make jokes and enjoy a bit of banter.
> **I am happy when:** I have someone to talk to and something to keep my hands busy.
> **You can help me by:** Listening to my stories.

The Three Strangers

Suad Aldarra

(1)

I did not realise how serious my father's condition was until he locked himself in the bathroom. When I arrived home in the evening, I sensed the air was different. The extra pairs of shoes behind the door told me we had visitors. I could hear my mother's sobbing and thick voices yelling in the living room. I raced through the long hallway of our house, my heart thumping wildly. My mother was sitting with her face buried in her hands while our neighbour Miss Huda tried, and failed, to calm her down. My brothers and some other neighbours stood in front of the bathroom door, knocking loudly. They were trying to reason with the person inside, my father.

'She wants to hurt me!'

I stood frozen in front of the locked door listening to my father's desperate yells.

My mother wept as she repeated over and over, *'Jann el rejjal!'* – the man has gone mad!

Turning to the neighbours, she asked, 'Is this my reward for taking care of him? I was just trying to bathe him.'

'He'd be lost without you,' Miss Huda said sympathetically, patting her shoulder.

The bell rang. I snapped out of my shocked state to answer the door. My uncle Sameer rushed in. He went straight to the bathroom. Someone must have filled him in. He pushed through the men blocking his way and started knocking heavily on the door.

'Abu Ahmad.' He put his ear on the door. 'It's me, Sameer. Open up for God's sake.'

'Is she out there?' My father's voice trembled like a kid hiding from ghosts.

'No, no ... we sent her away.' He waved his hand in the direction of my mother. 'Don't worry. I've got you.'

A few seconds later, the door finally cracked open and my father's skinny face appeared in the gap. His white underwear was the only thing covering his shaking body. Uncle Sameer reached for his hand and led him to the bedroom. As they walked slowly down the hallway he tried to talk to my father, reminding him how much my mother cared for him. After some long minutes, my father fell quiet and stopped arguing back. When I peeked into the bedroom, I saw my father. He was looking guilty. Later, Uncle Sameer helped him to finish his bath and put him down to rest in his own bed.

I squeeze my brain for a hidden memory. When did this start? When did my father begin to disappear in front of our eyes? When did he lose all that weight and when did his hand start shaking as he grabbed his teacup in the evening? It feels like yesterday that we sat together, casually allying up against my mother. My father liked to joke around. He refused to take life seriously. My mother was different. Every passing fly bothered her. She had to take responsibility for everything around the house while he enjoyed sitting back and living in the moment.

'When you get married, my dear Salwa,' my father would say, 'I'll dance *dabkeh* all night at your wedding.' His eyes sparkled with love.

My elder brother and sister got married, one after the other leaving the house, while I – the unexpected 'mistake' – stayed with my parents. I was unsure how to move on. My father's company was not only comfortable and warm, but safe. And I couldn't be sure I'd find that anywhere else.

Time stole tiny pieces of my father, slowly and quietly like a professional thief. One week he started to forget whether he'd prayed, so he double-prayed every time to rest his doubts. The following week, he took longer than usual returning from the mosque. The week after, he became furious with my mother, asking why she'd moved the bread. He couldn't find it anywhere. Once, he came home with a bruised knee and a cut on his forehead, leaning on a stranger who'd found him resting against the wall of the mosque, a few blocks away.

'Did you forget how to walk?' my mother said sarcastically as she cleaned his wound. She announced firmly that he wasn't allowed to go out alone anymore. It wasn't safe for him to go wandering round Damascus in the state he was in. This announcement didn't land well with my father.

Whenever we had visitors, there was a common game they liked to play with my father: Guess who it is? My father sometimes played along, guessing the names associated with the faces in his house. When he got an answer wrong everyone laughed, himself included sometimes. I tried to protect him from the embarrassment by giving him tips. I'd whisper the answer if the opportunity arose. My family would stare and hush me if they caught me doing this.

When Adnan proposed, or rather when his mother proposed, I was sitting there silent, blushing and shy in my family's house. I'd watched her sip her Turkish coffee slowly as she praised her precious son, all the time suspecting what was about to happen. I was genuinely shy. I was not pretending shyness for tradition's sake. I was thirty-three years old and had never looked a strange man in the eye. Adnan was wearing a grey suit and a seductive cologne. All the butterflies rushed in my stomach. I was charmed by the serious look of him, his well-shaved face and polite smile, the way he spoke in perfect sentences. My heart was juvenile back then. I knew Adnan was fifteen years older than me, divorced and living in Saudi Arabia, but these things didn't seem like a big deal. Everyone around me said I was lucky to have a suitor come knocking on the door at my age. I was well into my thirties after all. And I truly believed it too. I was lucky.

In the morning, I poured cups of coffee for my father and me. We sat on the balcony watching my beloved city wake up. Damascus looked peaceful at that time of the day, before its roads began bustling with traffic and car horns. My father held his smile as he sipped from his coffee. When I asked him about Adnan, he put his cup on the tray and looked straight at me like the wisest man on earth. Like he wasn't forgetful or confused anymore.

'It's your call, my sweet daughter. But I want to make sure you are safe with a man before I die. This society doesn't go easy on an unmarried woman.'

I felt the tears rushing to my eyes and a pull in my stomach. I was like a four-year-old girl at the school gate, holding tightly to her father's hand. *I don't want to leave you, Daddy*. I couldn't bring myself to say the words and he became distracted by an angry driver blowing his horn beneath our balcony. When he looked back at me, he asked me about my siblings – when were we going to school? I realised he was gone once again, like a beautiful sunset. I couldn't wait for him to rise again.

After two weeks, I said yes. Adnan and I became husband and wife. My father didn't get to dance at my wedding because we didn't have one. Adnan was in a rush to get back to Mecca. Besides, he'd already had an enormous wedding with his ex-wife. 'And look how that turned out,' he said by means of an excuse. He convinced me that a small party at my parents' house would be more intimate and less confusing for my father. Of course, I agreed. I would do anything for my father.

As I sat next to Adnan on the big couch in my parents' house, surrounded by my aunts and uncles, my eyes rested on my father. He looked happy, chatting with guests. I'd done the right thing. I repeated this silently, like a prayer. My father came over. I welcomed him with a stretched-out smile, proud to have his presence on my special day. But when he nodded curtly at Adnan without smiling, my heart began to tremble. He leaned in closer to whisper in my ear, 'I'm going out with my friends. I can't stand that guy sitting next to you.' I felt sick to my stomach. I hadn't done the right thing. Now it was too late.

My mother cried during the party, and every time I phoned her afterwards, she seemed like she had never stopped.

(2)

My lovely, handsome, well-spoken, good-smelling, mature new husband showed his true face shortly after we left Damascus. Had his eyes always been that angry and I'd just failed to notice before? I unpacked all my bright-coloured dresses and suits. Like every bride-to-be, I'd enjoyed putting my wardrobe together during our engagement. I soon realised I would only be allowed to wear black in this deserted part of the world. I still had to wear my vivid clothes at night. My new husband liked to have me look nice for him. When he arrived home late from yet another long day at work, he'd unlock the house door and then unlock me. It was painful in the beginning. It continued to be, but it hurt less than the loneliness.

Once a month I was allowed a long-distance phone call to my family. He'd sit next to me and watch my words like a human lie detector. The first time I said something he didn't approve of, he cut off the line and hid the phone somewhere in the house. He also read my letters before posting them. After he'd ripped the first two into shreds, I learnt what to write and what to bury deep inside me. Over time I worked out how to write letters like a happy wife. And when we visited home in summer, I mastered how to smile politely; the same way he'd smiled when he proposed.

My mother knew something was wrong the first time she looked me in the eye, but she told me the first year of marriage is always challenging and did not ask anything more. When I was reunited with my father, I couldn't drag myself out of his presence. I cried, my tears leaving damp patches on his shoulder. It was good to be back in his safe embrace. I wanted to say, *It's been a hell of a year, Daddy,* but I couldn't tell him. Adnan's stares were burning into my back, and my father was looking skinnier and more lost than before. He was so confused he kept praising Adnan all the time. I liked to think that this was my father's way of reminding Adnan he needed to step up and be the gentleman he pretended to be. He didn't seem to remember how he'd felt about my husband before and I couldn't tell if he believed what he was saying now or was lost in one of his absences. It didn't matter much. His kind words only made Adnan's ego grow bigger. He grew more and more cruel towards me, believing there would be no consequences to his actions.

Adnan gave me three children: Ashraf, Ameera, Ameer. He chose all their names, making sure they matched the first letter of his name. When I suggested Omar instead of Ashraf, because it was my favourite name for a little boy, I got a slap in the face. 'Is that your lover's name?' I was six months pregnant at the time. I never bothered suggesting names for the twins Ameera and Ameer. I knew better by then.

Five years after my marriage, my father passed away on a cold winter night. I missed his last days because Adnan wouldn't allow an unchaperoned trip back home and he couldn't take any time off work. 'He is already dead, so what's the rush for?'

My brother and sister filled me in about Abu Ahmad's final moments, how he faded away as he took his last breaths.

He'd asked for me over and over. They'd lied to him, insisting I was on my way. Adnan did not permit me to return home until later that summer. My mother gave me a copy of my father's death announcement printed on A4 paper. His name was written in the middle under the names of all the men who were related to him. According to tradition, no women were listed; not even my mother.

My father had become a paper. It was only then that I actually believed he was gone forever and let myself weep.

Life changed once I had kids. They gave me hope. I gave them cooked meals and clean clothes while Adnan bought them stuff: expensive and unnecessary stuff. We tried to pretend we were a normal, happy family. We muddled through for quite a few years until the kids became teenagers and wanted more than stuff and food on the table. They blamed me and Adnan for not loving them enough. I couldn't have loved those children more, but I couldn't say it in words or hugs. I didn't have enough words or hugs. When they started acting out against their father, I played the good wife. I always made sure to discipline them. A father should be respected no matter what. Later, they started yelling just like their father would yell at me, and I forgave them as I did with him.

When my kids were not kids anymore, one after the other they managed to escape their unloving home. They went to college and learnt how to be loved by other people. Soon it was Adnan and I, alone again.

Adnan was at work the first time he lost his balance and fell. His colleagues helped him up. One drove him home. The second time, he was in the house. The fall hurt his ankle, so he started using a stick to balance himself when he walked. The third fall landed him in the hospital. He was unconscious for some time. After scans and tests, the doctor confirmed he'd survived a stroke and might not be able to return to his previous everyday life.

The kids refused to come back to visit. Ameera told me over the phone, 'You chose to stay with that monster, now it looks like he's going to ruin your life in sickness as well as in health.' I couldn't believe the way they'd abandoned him. They simply opted out of caring for him at his worst. If only I'd had that option.

Adnan rejected the physiotherapy which could have helped him to walk again. He surrendered to his fate and stayed in bed while I patiently fed him, flipped the TV channels, changed his diapers and remained his prisoner. *How could I leave? What would people say if I left a sick man to die?* I wondered if I were sick what Adnan would do. This thought was even scarier than facing up to my present circumstances. I cared for Adnan. I thought of my reward in the afterlife. I did all the things I wished I could have done for my late father. This monster didn't deserve my kindness, but there was something satisfying about watching him lie there, weak and small.

Adnan asked for his mother continuously. Sometimes he'd called me Mother and I'd wonder who he was seeing when he looked at me. He woke me up at night, demanding to know why we were still here, not there, not home. He asked to see the kids who were not kids anymore; the kids who didn't want to see him again.

I was relieved that Adnan couldn't hurt me anymore. Maybe it was God's plan to keep him suffering so he could atone for his sins before he died. But when was he ever going to die?

Astaghfer Alla – forgive me, God.

When I texted Ameera about God's plan, she told me to stop making excuses for Adnan and Allah. She had gone astray so I prayed for her. I blamed myself for letting her go, for letting all my children go.

(3)

The window curtains dance back and forth, allowing sporadic threads of sunshine to fall upon a picture on the wall. It's a photograph of a man and a woman and three children. I am lying in bed, mesmerised, hypnotised. I know that picture. That's Baba and Mama and my siblings. I smile and think of Eid's sweets and the toys we were given when we went to have this family portrait taken.

I don't know how much time passes before I become aware of the strange man sitting on a chair next to my bed. His fingers separate the pages of a book he's clutching in his hand. His eyes are familiar like a song I used to sing all the time and then, one day, forgot about.

'Abu Ahmad?'

He smiles, half a smile. His eyes are now watery.

'No, *Mama*, it's me. Ashraf.' He places his warm hand in mine and kisses it gently. I am terrified but then he adds, 'your son'.

Ashraf is tall and handsome, a replica of my father. I warm up a little, responding to his concerned look and tender touch. I paste a smile on my face and nod. I know this man.

'Did you like what I just read?' Ashraf turns the book in his hand to show me the cover. I read a name slowly. *Is that my name? Did I write that book?*

'This is your book, Mama. It was a big hit back in 2022.'

I move my gaze between the book and Ashraf. I can't understand. *Did I write a book?* Ashraf looks at me for a long time without saying a word. He then stands up and puts the book on the busy bookcase which stands next to my family portrait. My gaze once more falls upon the faces. *Wait. That's not Mama. That's me. And that's little Ashraf, with the twins.* Fear grips me. *Adnan. Why is Adnan there?* I try to get out of bed, but I can't move a muscle. Ashraf notices. He follows my gaze to the photograph as I repeat Adnan's name in horror. He rushes to rescue me.

'It's ok Mama. You are ok. Baba is not here anymore.'

He arranges the duvet on top of me and kisses me on the forehead.

'I'll never understand why you decided to stay with him until the end but he's gone, Mama, slowly and painfully like Ameera wished.'

Ashraf's face is a mix of sadness, sorrow and anger. For a moment he looks like he's about to hit the wall, then his expression softens. 'We were all reborn after his death. Remember, you turned all those secret writings that you'd kept over the years into a book. And the twins are fine. They're travelling the world and looking after each other, and I found a warm, loving woman who taught me how to love unconditionally.' Ashraf's face lights up with a smile as he lifts the photo down from the wall and carries it over to my bed. 'You know that's not Baba in the picture,' he says, his finger pointing out each person in turn. 'That's me, Mama. And that's Zainab, my wife, Rami, Susan and little Salwa.' His smile grows bigger. 'She is kind and sweet, just like you.'

I look at the picture again and I see the same guy standing in front me posing happily with his arm draped round a woman's shoulders and three kids standing next to them. My heart feels warm but my mind is a battlefield.

'I'll come again tomorrow and bring them with me,' Ashraf says. 'Rest well now, Mama.'

He turns to leave the room as a lady wearing a loose pink top and pants comes in. She says it's time for bed. I'm already in bed, but I don't bother correcting her. I close my eyes and search desperately for my father's faded image in the darkness. I see him. I feel his embrace. My heartbeats slow down like the end of a song. I am safe now.

A New Day, Tomorrow

Henrietta McKervey

I wake, immediately sure that I've had a good – a really good – sleep.

The type babies have, swaddled and cocooned with nothing troubling their soft, empty heads ... and definitely without the sore knees and regrets that sting me awake night after night. It's the best sleep I've had in years.

Keeping my eyes shut, I turn my head slightly. The pillowcase is soft yet crisp, and smells faintly of lavender. Real lavender, not that fake stuff that stinks like a pub toilet. The duvet is a perfect weight too, just heavy enough to feel warm, yet light enough that I'm not sweating. I've been plagued by night sweats for years, waking chilly and early, damp streaks underwiring my boobs. 'Ah, Mammy,' Juliet said only recently, 'you can't still be menopausal, not ten years later! It's called the change, not the permanent.' 'Wait till it's your turn,' I told her, 'you won't be such a smarty-pants then.' But she just threw her eyes up to heaven.

I shift slightly onto my side and fart gently, enjoying the soft touch of the mattress when I lower my right buttock back down. I've all the time in the world, I tell myself, imagining lying flaked out on a cloud, drifting across an empty blue sky with nothing else to do but trail the horizon. I picture myself striking a godlike pose, all toga and cotton-wool beard, torso rising through the cloud, with one hand on either side of its fluffy, yet surprisingly substantial, edges.

My entire body feels light and cleansed, rather than washed, if you see what I mean: as if my overworked, neglected insides had been valeted overnight. It reminds me of the first hours after Juliet was born and that glorious sensation – no, more than that, the certainty – of being empty again. Of being still and alone and separate, finally. You're not meant to think of the baby inside you as a parasite, but once the thought lands it's hard to shake. Poor Juliet! If she'd only had a baby herself, she'd understand.

Finally, I open my eyes, but I don't recognise a thing. I'm in a bed, yes. But it's not my bed. There's a door where the door is in my room at home, and the corner window is just like I have at home, but it's not my window. The curtains are the same, but definitely newer, brighter. Cleaner too, if I'm honest. Where is this? What's happening? My stomach begins to churn. I can feel panic rising. I look at my hands clutching the duvet cover. My fingers are shaking, spotted and ugly against the soft fabric. Everything in this room – this lovely, warm, terrifying room – is white. Where am I? I wonder, suddenly afraid tears will flood my eyes.

Maybe I'm a ghost? Why on earth am I thinking this? It's the sense of weightlessness, I realise, as though my body is disappearing. You see, I believe that we are always falling apart. That sounds desperately grim, but I don't see it that way. For me, it's the truth, the secret heart of all the things we care about and worry about and remember and forget: everything is disappearing, bit by bit. The day I realised this was like exhaling properly for the first time. Go on, try it; admit you are slipping away. Your life will thank you for it.

I'm pretty sure I'm not a ghost. Of course, that doesn't mean I'm alive either. Perhaps I'm dead? Mother of divine, please tell me I'm not in heaven. I've always thought heaven would be a very dull place, all *no-no-please-after-you* and *sure-whatever-you're-having-yourself*. I've spent my life trying to chivvy people's spirits along, keeping the peace. If heaven is more of that, you can stick it.

'No,' a woman's voice interrupts my thoughts. I hadn't noticed her come in the door, nor realised I'd spoken aloud. 'No,' she says again, 'you're not dead.' She stands beside my bed, smiling. 'You're not in hell either,' she says. She's not laughing at me – her face is kind – but I feel like a child, unsure what options are left. Purgatory, that medieval Ponzi scheme, doesn't count, though I think limbo was worse; a tax on the hopes of the living. If heaven and hell, good and bad are ruled out, what's left? I've often wondered have I been too binary? Have I reduced everything to yes/no, happy/sad?

Maybe I'm as good as dead, I think. I'm immediately cross with myself, because I've heard people say that about my brother Maurice and it always annoys me. I'm too young to be dead. I'm only sixty-one. And I've been feeling grand. Not sick or anything, though I know that doesn't mean much, considering the speed at which death comes for some people. I'm fine compared to some of my friends and my husband Eddie. I'm certainly in a better state than Maurice.

'You're frowning,' the woman says. From behind her back she produces a tray, pivoting on one foot like a dancer.

'Who are you?' I say. 'If you don't mind me asking,' I add.

'Hiya.'

'Hiya, to you too,' I reply, seriously unsure what's going on, but not wanting to be rude. I never want to be rude. I used to think of it as a superpower: Princess Polite! As I got older, my good manners began to feel more like a bag of rocks I was lugging around, entirely useless and forever weighing me down.

'No,' she says. 'H-A-L-I-A. My name.' She gestures to a name badge pinned below her shoulder. She is wearing white scrubs, her style more that of a beautician than a surgeon. The badge and outfit mean I'm in a place where staff wear uniforms. I run through other uniforms in my mind, which makes me think of *Find Your Place!*, the handbook our career guidance teacher Miss Cantwell passed around the class the year we finished secondary school. Nurse, air hostess, chambermaid ... you can imagine. Actually, *Find Your Place!* didn't include any chambermaids. It should have, if only to warn me off spending a hot, tearful summer in London slaving in a cheap hotel across the road from Victoria Station, the Jif permanently to hand, ready to squirt the day porter when he tried to put himself between me and the door of the cleaning press. Scrubbing and tidying ten hours a day in a city stinking of rotting dustbins and strangers.

God, I haven't thought of Miss Cantwell – Miss Cantshite, we called her – in decades. Each girl got one private conversation with her. 'Turns,' she called them. We didn't get appointments, or meetings. We got turns. My school's only attempt in six years to have a conversation with me about my future took less than ten minutes. Miss Cantwell kept her left hand in her cardigan pocket the entire time. I could see the outline of her fingers wrapped around a packet of fags, her index finger tapping the cardboard. 'I can see you doing something in a uniform,' she said, narrowing her eyes. 'Hmm,' she said, agreeing with herself. She looked me up and down as if she was a judge with a dozen ponies in front of her and only a single rosette to hand out. 'Hmmm,' she said again. 'Have you thought about the bank?' The bank! Me! The memory makes me giggle.

'Are you okay, Jenny?'

'I am Halia, thanks. But tell me, where am I?'

'Where do you think you are?'

'I'm too comfortable to be at home, I can tell you that much.'

'Food is only served in the dining room,' she says.

Had I asked her for something to eat? I don't think so.

'But, you know, as you're new ...' she trails off, a conspiratorial grin finishing the sentence.

Ah ha! I think. So I *am* somewhere new! It's strange I don't remember arriving, but I'm canny, I'll find a way. Halia smiles again and my previous unease dissipates, an early mist melting away. Instead, I have the most lovely calm sensation. And even though the unusualness of the feeling makes me wonder if being relaxed isn't my natural state, Halia's smile is so soothing I don't feel any urgency to do anything.

'Why not sit up and have something to eat?' she says. 'You slept through breakfast and lunch. I've got a super dinner for you.'

I wriggle into a sitting position, the pillows repositioning themselves behind my back with only the barest nudge from my elbow. She puts the tray down on my lap. Chicken in a cream sauce with a big scoop of mash and a big heap of mushrooms. I lean down and sniff the plate.

'There's plenty of thyme,' Halia says.

I nod, delighted with the delicious herby smell. Maurice used to make creamy lemon thyme chicken with spuds and mushrooms fried in butter. I taste a forkful. It tastes exactly as his always did. He was – no, is, I remind myself– a fabulous chef. Just because he is no longer able to cook doesn't mean his skills never existed.

She smiles. 'Thyme,' she says again. 'I'll be back when it's thyme.' I look at my plate, confused again.

'T-I-M-E,' she says.

'Right you are,' I reply. I've no clue what she means. But, do you know what? I don't care. 'This is the business,' I say as I tuck in. There's a small silver dish with three dark chocolates arranged like a shamrock and a pot of coffee with the plunger already pressed down. 'You'll be dishwater,' I say to myself, but when I pour a cup, it's perfect.

'You did well,' Halia now says, reaching for the tray. I hadn't noticed her come back into the room. 'But you look tired now.' And do you know what? As she says it, I begin to think maybe I am, maybe I am. 'Why not have a snooze?' she suggests. 'We've loads of time.' There she goes again. Some people are obsessed with time. I used to think I never had enough. And then I had so much, I'd have given it away if I could. Run the tap until the tank was dry.

I close my eyes and snuggle down, full of dinner. As I'm dozing off, an aspirin ad that used to be on TV comes into my head. Years ago, this was. A woman dressed in an office rigout (no uniform for her!) with an open trench coat is struggling up the stairs to her flat. She has blonde hair in a straggly end-of-the-day bun – well, TV straggly, which means pretty with wisps, not greasy and collapsing around her ears, like in real life. She's struggling under the weight of a big bag of shopping and is carrying a red-haired toddler who's having a conniption, when the heel of her shoe snaps off. Her expression suggests that her first thought is to toss the child over the bannisters. Instead, she lugs the lot into her flat, takes an aspirin, and all's well again. The toddler is laughing. Her shopping has mysteriously disappeared into the kitchen cupboards. She looks delighted with herself.

I used to think about that ad a lot when Juliet was young. The pretty office lady, rushing home, her angry child in her arms. You're not meant to take tablets for longer than a few days according to the packet, so the aspirin was never going to be a long-term solution. Perhaps it was the office job she needed to give up? Or maybe move to a flat on the ground floor? Taking a tablet wouldn't make her husband do the messages instead of her, or collect the ginger whinger. If anything, that ad showed how rubbish aspirin is. It wouldn't help her at all.

'Yeah, I hear you,' Halia says.

I must have been telling her about the ad. 'Sorry,' I say. 'Do I go on a bit? I don't mean to.'

'Not at all,' she says. 'Do you think the woman represents an intersection of third-wave feminism with unjust societal pressures masquerading as self-determined expectations of working women?'

'Ah yeah,' I say. 'Plus, you know, getting people to buy aspirin.'

'How about that nap now?' she asks and I snuggle down again, only delighted with myself.

***

I wake, immediately sure I've had a good, a really good, sleep.

I've never felt so comfortable. The duvet is a perfect weight, just heavy enough to feel warm yet light. The touch of it is comforting, familiar, and there's a faint smell I can't place. Fabric softener, is it? I make a note to ask … what was her name? I crash around the filing cabinets of my mind. Halia, that's it.

'Hello,' she says, appearing inside the room, like before. Her left arm is by her side yet her right hand is up by her ear, the first two fingers high and bent as if holding an invisible lit cigarette.

'You're some woman,' I tell her. 'It's like you can tell I'm thinking about you.' In my mouth is the faint taste of chicken, and I remember the mash and mushrooms, just like Maurice used to make. 'That dinner earlier was the business.'

'It was yesterday. You slept for fourteen hours.'

'I did not!'

'You did. People often do when they arrive. There's a lot to take in, it's tiring. And today is going to be a busy day, so I thought you'd be glad of the rest. Do you remember this?' she asks, unfolding a large square of fabric. She holds it wide and flaps it like a bullfighter, and I'm tempted to jump out of bed and run towards her, my fingers pointed into horns.

'No,' I say, crestfallen, as if I've failed a test I didn't know I was taking. 'I don't think so

'Maurice gave it to you,' she says. The fabric, which is silk, has a pattern of red and violet flowers and dappled green leaves. The flowers bend and sway in her hands, twisting on their shining stalks. I remember now. I'd spotted it in Marks & Spencer's years ago when Maurice and I were in town for lunch in the rooftop café (no better man for a hot counter), but I hadn't bought it. He'd said I should, that it was very flattering and sure wouldn't the cost-per-wear end up next to nothing. I still hadn't bought it. I'd regretted it after and went back the following week, only it was gone. And then on my birthday he'd presented it to me, still in the M&S bag with the receipt at the bottom. He'd bought it when I was in the toilet.

Maurice was my best friend, which has always mattered more than him being my brother. Best friends sounds like something kids say, doesn't it? But it's true. He was. I can't say he is, because our friendship doesn't exist in the present tense anymore even though our relationship does. But he was, he really was.

'Maurice doesn't remember me,' I say.

'That's why you're here,' Halia says. 'Come with me,' she adds and I don't need telling twice. She leads me into a circular room, lined with doors yet empty of furniture. A strange room. It has a Sunday-afternoon-movie quality to it. You know the sort of film where the set is expensive but the dialogue's cheap? 'Wait here,' she says. 'I'll be back in a minute.'

One of the doors opens and a man enters.

'Hello Auntie Jenny,' he says. 'It's me: Andy!'

'Are you sure?' I ask, confused.

When Rosie – the witch Maurice married by mistake – left him, she took their little lad Andy to Glasgow. He was six. Maurice only got to see him a couple of times a year. Rosie made it so hard. I'll never forgive her for that. Three years later, Andy got septicaemia and died. It brought Maurice so low. I think he'd assumed it would all work out in time, that Andy knew his dad loved him, that their separation was a long exhalation and one day they'd breathe in again. He talked about Andy a lot for the first year or so after his death, then barely spoke of him at all, as if what was binding his throat had slowly tightened like a noose. It was a terrible, terrible business. I'd use other words if I had them, but I don't. Language is like that. It lets you down when you need it most. You look for the words but they're gone, leaving craters in the surface where they've been spooned out.

Immediately I worry that Andy will think I'm accusing him of lying.

'I'm sorry Andy, love,' I say, 'but I haven't seen you since you were six. And, I don't want to be rude, but how can you be an adult? You died when you were nine.'

'I grew up,' he tells me.

'Here?' I wonder, looking around the room of doors.

'No, in Dad's imagination. This is who I am now.'

'You turned out great,' I say. And it's true; he's incredibly handsome. Andy was a lovely little lad, but he was no looker. 'Have you a job?'

He nods. 'I'm a doctor,' he says. 'A paediatric anaesthetist. I was a bank manager for a long time, but when Dad lost his savings during the bank collapse, he decided I'd be better off as a doctor.'

'Great decision,' I say. 'Being a doctor must keep you busy.'

'It does,' he nods again. 'Though I always make time to volunteer with the homeless too.'

'Your father would be as proud as punch,' I say. 'And have you a family of your own?' And what do you know … of course he does! Two girls, two boys. 'Ah, that's lovely, Andy,' I tell him. And I mean it, because I know Maurice would have loved grandchildren. He'd have been great with them.

Andy takes a picture from his pocket. The image is quite blurry, but from what I can make out, the four little faces all look very like him as a kid.

'It's not a great shot, sure it's not?'

He looks at the picture as if he'd never really considered it before. 'Little imps,' he says. 'Sure, they never stay still long enough to get their picture taken.'

'Andy!' Halia is back by my side. 'How did you get in here?' she asks, making a vamoose gesture with her hand. His face crumples. He suddenly looks six again and lost, the way he used to look in the months before his mother took him away. I remember him as a happy little boy, then a worried-looking lad, then absent, then … well, then nothing. A disjointed sequence of memories strung together by photographs. Looking sheepish, he leaves, shutting the white door behind him.

'Bye-bye, Andy love!' I call out after him. He doesn't look back.

'Sorry, that shouldn't have happened,' Halia says and I nod. Really though, how would I know? I haven't a breeze what's happening. 'It was nice to see how well Andy turned out for Maurice, all the same,' I tell her.

Halia touches a door. It opens onto a laneway. We don't step through, we just watch a girl and boy, maybe four and nine, playing together. It's me, I realise. Me and Maurice, behind the house we grew up in. It was a shared laneway behind the terrace, a world of kids and dustbins. We're oddly black and white though, and jerky, like Pathé newsreel footage.

'What's that about?' I ask. 'We're not that old!'

'Sorry,' Halia goes, 'contrast troubles.'

She takes a remote control from the pocket of her scrubs and presses a few buttons. That's more like it. We're in colour again, normal-looking. Maurice's left knee is scraped. I remember that morning now. I had just pushed him against a wall for no reason, just because no one was looking and I so rarely had any sort of advantage against my older, bigger brother. His knee had scraped the length of a rough brick. While I'm watching him rub the blood away, we turn monochrome again.

'Sorry,' Halia says. 'Probably a short circuit. 'I'll lodge a ticket with the technical team.'

Another door opens. Maurice and me are having supper in our pyjamas, sitting by the fire with our hair still damp. We're reading comics: *The Beezer* for him, *Twinkle* for me. 'That'd be a Saturday night,' I tell Halia. 'Bath night.' He is looking at his favourite strip, The Numskulls, which is about tiny people who live in your brain and control your mind and movements. I loved The Numskulls too. Their existence made more sense to me as a child than any description of how my body really worked.

She opens another door and here we are again, years later. I'm still in my school uniform but Maurice is in brand new painter's whites. He must have just started his apprenticeship. We're sitting on a wall, and he's letting me have a drag on his cigarette. Another door and we're sitting in a pub in Dun Laoghaire after Rosie has gone. Maurice looks sad and lost and drunk. He stares at me, his expression glazed. Another and we're at the greyhounds. Maurice rips up a betting slip and my husband Eddie slags him for picking losers. Watching this now makes me scarlet, because it was only a few months after Rosie left. It didn't strike me at the time that Eddie was being insensitive, but he was. I watch a couple of Christmases, several birthdays, two holidays in Wexford and one in Spain. Door after door opens, until the room is spinning around me. I begin to experience a deep-set unease; an intense feeling of being homesick for a place I've never visited.

I watch Maurice on a building site, silent and tense as his boss Dermod Kelly berates him, every second word a fuck-this or shite-that, scattering expletives the way you'd shake salt over your dinner. It makes me angry to see my polite, orderly brother stand there, forced to absorb another man's foul-mouthed tirade. Finally, Kelly takes his own advice and fucks off. Maurice moves to one side and lights a cigarette. He has a gnawing, worried look on his face, an expression I know well; fear that the world might crack open and swallow him whole. The edges of this scene are tinged with purple, a sky turning ugly before a storm.

'I always suspected Kelly was a total prick,' I say.

'Yes,' Halia nods. 'He never comes out well.' She looks like she wants to say more but stops herself. 'We're not meant to comment on anyone's memories,' she explains. 'Sorry, I shouldn't have said anything.'

'You don't need to,' I tell her. 'A prick's a prick.'

'You'll like this one,' she says, and walks to a door with a warm glow of light spilling out from under it. Maurice is carrying a little girl on his back. It's Juliet, I realise and my heart leaps at the happy little head on her. Me and Eddie, our arms full of beach gear, are plodding ahead of them through a sand dune, our footsteps heavy and tired. Juliet is wearing a sunhat and singing 'Somewhere Over the Rainbow' in Maurice's ear, her arms like a scarf around his neck.

She pauses and asks, 'Would you like to be the rain, Uncle Momo?'

'No,' he replies. 'I want to be the sea. The biggest wave in the biggest ocean.'

'I'll be rain, so I can rain on your wave and make it even bigger,' she says.

'Great idea,' he tells her. 'You're a genius!'

'I love you, Momo,' she says.

He tightens his grip under her legs. 'I love you too,' he says, then adds, 'what's your name again?'

She hoots with laughter. I watch myself walking ahead of them, glancing back only once, quickly, and frowning at them.

'You know where you are now, don't you?' Halia asks. 'You're in Maurice's imagination. This place is called the Memory Keep.'

'What?'

'It's where he is most alive.'

'I'm inside his brain?' I can hear the incredulity in my voice. Which is fair enough, because what she's just said is ridiculous. She reads my mind again.

'No, the Memory Keep is the least ridiculous thing there is, if you think about it,' she says. 'You don't think your memories are just your own, do you? Where did you think shared memories go?'

'Wait,' I say, suddenly thinking of something. 'Andy!' I say, not quite keeping the *so-there* tone out of my voice. 'How can he be a memory if he didn't exist?'

'That's where the imagination comes in,' she says. 'For Maurice, memory and imagination are not so much colliding as mingling. Remember how blurred Andy's kids were in the photo? It's not that they wouldn't pose properly, it's that they were never fully there; never properly realised.'

Despite how crazy this sounds, it makes sense too. Maurice had imagined himself a grown-up son (who must have cost him an imaginary fortune in imaginary college fees), so perhaps giving Andy a relationship and kids as well was just too much. Stretching out a nine year old he'd barely seen in three years – with thick glasses and hair so curly around his head it was like he'd been knitted – into an adult was probably enough of a task without imagining his missus and four – four! – little ones. Still, fair play for trying Maurice, for forcing your way through such uncommon sorrow.

'I don't think I should be here,' I tell her. 'This doesn't seem right to me.' I feel like I'm smearing my fingerprints all over Maurice's memories, pawing at his imagination. His memories are private, they're his. 'Plus,' I add, 'they're different to mine.'

I'm thinking of Juliet and him laughing on the beach, while I walked ahead, oblivious to their conversation.

'Oh, we take ethics very seriously,' Halia says. 'Remind me to give you the leaflet. You will only see the memories in which you feature.'

'What about the prick?'

'Maurice was thinking about you while Dermod Kelly was shouting at him.'

'I don't want his memories,' I say, suddenly hot and angry. 'I don't want to be in his imagination. I want *him* back, in my present, not my past.'

'That's not possible. Isn't this better than nothing?'

'So this whole place ... it's only *his* imagination?'

She shakes her head. 'The Memory Keep is open to anyone, but it's zoned to avoid mix-ups. We have an application process. It's very straightforward. No one is turned away.'

'You do this sort of thing,' I gesture pointlessly around, at the walls, the doors, 'with lots of people?'

'Yes, I have a very busy caseload at the moment.'

'Does he know I'm here?'

Halia smiles her lovely smile. 'He has to want it to happen, that's how the Memory Keep works.'

And what if I didn't want to be here, I'm about to say. Before I can speak there's a sudden noise, like a storm blasting outside. The walls begin to shake. The doors fly open and slam shut, over and over, loud and angry.

'Maurice is upset,' Halia says. My knees buckle under me and I fall to the floor. The lights crackle and the room goes dark.

'Halia?' I cry out.

'It's alright,' she says, as the lights come back on. 'It's alright, he's calming down. You must be exhausted. How about a lie-down? We can talk more tomorrow.'

'I'll still be here?'

'If you want to stay, you will wake up here. If you don't, you won't.'

She leads me back to my white room and tucks me into bed. She pats the duvet smooth. What a kind woman she is, I think.

'Thanks,' she says.

'I don't know how you do that, but it's very impressive,' I murmur as I begin to doze off, picturing Maurice's memory of him and Juliet walking to the beach. It was so different to my own recollection of that afternoon. Eddie and I had walked ahead because we were scrapping and I didn't want Juliet to overhear us. If anyone were to ask me, I would say yes, my husband and I have always been happy, ordinary and happy, yet that day Eddie had annoyed me, or I had annoyed him … who knows what it was about. It didn't matter, then or now. My recollection of that moment is that Eddie and I were overheated, pinked-up and cranky, not yet adjusted to the unfamiliar pattern of a holiday. I'd glanced behind me just once, my arms laden and tired, ready to get snippy with Maurice if he and Juliet were lagging too far behind us.

'See you in the morning,' Halia says. She gently closes the door behind her. I lie perfectly still. Tomorrow, will I wake, immediately sure I've had a good, a really good, sleep? Do I want to explore the world moving underneath my brother's memories; a place of subterranean vaults and blacked-out caves, of shade and cool light, of shadows and scorch marks?

I keep my eyes shut tight, and concentrate again until I can smell sea salt, warm sand, and the faint tang of sandwich cream from the picnic bag I was carrying that long-gone day. I listen closely to the past until I can hear the slap of my flip-flops against the path, and the breezy crackle of the dry grass lining the sand dunes. I tell Eddie to be quiet, that we can argue later. That we've the rest of our lives to fight, if we want to. I turn my memory-self around. The murmur of voices and laughter grows clearer. It's bright and giddy, rising above the crash of the waves. Juliet is singing! I hadn't heard it back then. I can hear it now. And Maurice, my dear, lost brother who no longer knows me, nor remembers the stretch of our days together, is happy; a man without fears or misgivings. I watch him as he squints into the sun, and I hear him join in her song, his voice thin and cracking and full of hope.

What, You Egg

Elaine Feeney

Your new room was next to the reception. You were moved when they found you floating in the bath. By then you had begun to sleep through visits and I sat there for hours listening to staff chatting through the paper-thin walls or staring through your window at the unambitious rockery and overgrown leylandii. In late June, a tiny rose tree bloomed. The rooms were small, connected to a bathroom covered with blue tiles to the ceiling; no curtain, no rail, only a shower now and a plug hole in the ground. Nothing left to end yourself. Not that that was ever your intention.

You love water, I said in your defence as they towel-dried your hair and inflated a blood pressure cuff on your arm. You've always wanted to jump in the sea, I continued in my habit of explaining another's actions. You had never been in the sea, but I was flustered rushing to be with you, imagining you soaked through your nightie to your purple-blue skin, the trails of silver stitch marks running up your legs where you'd had your veins done. Sat up in the bed, braless, as everything was hazardous to you. You were bewildered. The new room seemed strange without cushions, and your photographs and small yellow notes were gone.

In the early days I had promised to take you home on Tuesday. Always Tuesday. 'I'll take you home on Tuesday,' I'd say, 'just wait for the weekend, for some rest.'

'Promise?'

'Promise.'

I found your photographs and Post-its outside on a flowerpot by the bins. I put them back up but you got agitated, working too hard to remember faces, exhausting yourself rote-learning the messages off the squares of paper: where you worked, what you listened to on the radio, your favourite cake.

The permanent signs were the same: *Don't Touch, Press for Assistance. Hot Water. No Visitors After 9 p.m.*

You sat rigid as your wet hair fell in childish ringlets and your eyes were all bloodshot.

'Don't you just love water?' I said, talking to the silence.

The walls closed in by the late afternoon, so I took you out to sit in the dining room, though neither of us was hungry. The long hall full of wafts of cabbage and pork ribs, the tall windows draped with paisley curtains. Always the same vanilla ice cream, always red seats, always a fear of choking, always checking for bones, always someone running, always a woman sat opposite you with velvet slippers on the wrong feet, always the clock never ticking, its dead battery corroding the plastic battery slot behind the clock-face. Tea, always a mushroom omelette.

'Do you remember the eggs?' you said, as you waved a plastic spoon at me.

'No,' I said, lying. Always the same egg story.

'You know the woman in the scullery?' you said, waving the spoon quicker now.

'Your mother?'

'What, you? No, don't be so, so …' and then you stopped as though the wind had gone against you. Eventually you said, 'Some evening you might come over and sit outside and have wine in those goblet glasses Mrs Faye liked.'

I knew you didn't drink wine.

'You do remember Mrs Faye?'

I nodded.

'I wonder would Mrs Faye like a glass of wine?'

I nodded again.

'Well don't just sit there, get her some.'

And so, I got up and went back to your bedroom for a little while and sat on the lid of the toilet and stared at myself in your small mirror.

You never forgot Mrs Faye, even on days when you couldn't remember the word for love or dinner or bread or the fingers you stared at excitedly like a child discovering their digits for the first time. You followed their movement as they hinged forward at the knuckle. Your eyes were rolling after them, and losing your balance, you fell forwards onto the table. Bang. As I lifted you up by your narrow shoulders, you picked up my hands.

'They're nice,' you said, rubbing my fingers and twisting my wedding band about in circles. 'We were never allowed to wear rings in the bakery.'

*

When you first started in the bakery you worked the hot ovens all day. Mrs Faye sat up front by the huge glass counter filled with pastries and warm breads. She watched the girls with white aprons over black uniforms serve customers at the small café tables. When it was quiet, Mrs Faye walked about the huge kitchen down the back, fixing the layout of loaves on the wire rack as they cooled, making certain they didn't touch off one another.

Every day you walked home at lunchtime, dipping into the dark scullery for some toast and a quick chat with the woman stood by the sink washing Delft or scrubbing stains off children's clothes.

'"Don't forget the eggs," she'd say as you left.'

'Who'd say?' you said, pushing your finger into some vanilla ice cream and leaving a hollow thumb print. 'Who'd say?' you said again.

'The woman in the scullery,' I said.

'Ah, her,' you said, pulling my wedding ring off my finger and placing it into the hole in the ice cream. 'Yes, yes. Always looking for eggs that one, when she ran out of ...' And then you fell silent again, distracted by a toddler hiding behind the curtain who jumped out now and then, laughing loudly.

She was always worried, you said as you snapped the plastic spoon in half.

On evenings when there was no meat or fish in the house, your mother wanted eggs brought home from town after you'd clocked off. To feed the children before they went to sleep. Usually, she wanted eggs on evenings he was drinking. Evenings the house had nothing left to eat. End of week days, middle of week days. Your mother worked for Mrs Faye's father before you worked for Mrs Faye. You went to the same primary school. When your mother started to work for her father, she would swan into the shop. Even though she was just a young girl then, she'd been born with the manners of the world already formed. She'd bypassed the stupidity of childhood. The men in the kitchens lifted her up in a fuss and spun her about and she would swan back out through the shop after the attention, as though it was the most normal thing in the world to live so freely, taking a coin from the till, or a scone from the basket as she went. When primary school was over, she'd bring her friends by from the boarding school she attended. It was outside the city near Connemara and run by Benedictine nuns. They would sit chatting for hours at the small round café tables as your mother served them.

After your time on the bread ovens, you moved on to the pastry line. Mrs Faye allowed you to stay back after work to make pastry in the evenings, to feel its coldness, how quick it turned to crumbs, to figure out that moment just before it would crumble, the speed of a basic shortcrust, the laborious croquembouche, timings of what needed to be worked on the thick wooden plinths. *Practice,* you called it. It was more refined than working clumsy bread dough all day and you had the big kitchen to yourself. The older bakers, all men, had clocked off and gone up to Staunton's for pints before tea. Some skipped tea and came to work the next morning doubled over and sweating madly in the kitchen's heat. Most of the shop girls ran out at five, excitedly, as though they had somewhere to be. When the kitchen was empty, you could make your mistakes alone. No one noticed except the young boy from Eyre Street who mopped the floors in his bare feet. Mrs Faye stayed up front after the shop closed. She'd pull off her scarf, push away her court shoes from her feet and cash up. Sometimes she oiled the wooden tables, the wood drinking in the linseed oil, or she polished the skirting boards for hours on her hands and knees, drinking small café glasses of wine.

*

It was a bitter cold day for April.

You'd finished up work and were skipping pastry practice to get the eggs. After time was called, you'd gone out into the bakery's back yard to splash water from the huge tin sink under the eave onto your hot face. Returning inside, you stood by the coat hooks and lifted your heavy apron off your narrow body, revealing a papery white shirt. You hung the apron up onto the hook, where you would always hang your coat. But you had not brought your duffel coat today, as it was now April and you were optimistic about spring. School taught that spring was yellow flowers, lambs, powerful woman saints in the sunshine. Soon, summer would follow with time for the seaside. Maybe you would call in on Mary

Quin who you hadn't seen since you finished school. You were bursting to tell her that you worked the pastry station now. You went up to the front of the shop where Mrs Faye was chatting quickly as she served Dr Brown. You had not heard him come in. She was picking out two fruit scones.

'Weren't you lucky you just caught us?' Mrs Faye said to Dr Brown.

'Ah, you'd open up for me,' Brown said, winking, as she passed a paper bag over the high glass counter. He clutched it tight by the neck.

'And do you know what?' he said, pausing a minute, 'maybe grab me a cream horn for Sara.'

'She deserves spoiling,' Mrs Faye said, glancing about the empty cake trays. 'I have one in the fridge out the back. I'll only be a minute,' she called out as she scurried along the tiles and out to the back of the shop. 'She must be due any day now.'

'Yes. Yes. Due this week,' Brown shouted after her.

You stood there with the doctor, half coy, half fool under the big lights of the shop. Brown looked hard at you. First, he nodded approvingly at your shoes, and then moved his eyes upwards slowly along your body. You didn't dare lift the sole of your foot up off the floor. You were hiding the linoleum piece which sealed up a circular hole in the shoe sole. You blushed hot, his eyes now on your white shirt.

Mrs Faye rushed back in with the pastry held out like a torch, wrapped in a green serviette.

'You're in luck ...' she said, waving the horn and swinging herself back around the counter to wrap it up. But she watched him looking at you. And then she stared too and your face reddened more now. You looked down at your shoes as Mrs Faye dropped the pastry onto the tiles right by your toe.

'Damn it!' she said, and apologised. Brown quickly leaned over the mess on the floor, half-bowing forward, his herringbone coat flocking about his thin frame.

'No matter, Mrs Faye, let's just clean this up,' and he wiped the floor with the serviette. 'She's best without it in any case,' he said.

'You should be off now,' Mrs Faye said suddenly and began grabbing up the ends of his herringbone like a crazy bridesmaid fussing with swathes of a wedding dress. 'You just never know with your first,' she said, 'that baby could come anytime, off you go now. You really must go.'

Brown left with the bag clutched in a tight grip, his small finger with its ruby signet cocked outwards.

Mrs Faye turned the *Open* sign *Closed*, pushed up the bolts of the door, and spun about to face you.

'I'd expect nothing else from you,' she said, staring at your chest. 'To be frank,' she said, catching her breath, 'you make me ill.' Then she sidled back behind the glass counter, pulled a clutch of receipts to cash up. And everything was quiet for a moment as you stood there, trying to slow down your breath. Then suddenly, she turned about in a flash and was back outside the counter. She lifted her right hand and slapped you hard across the face.

*

Your heart was pumping fizzy blood now, the kind that disorientates you and makes it impossible to think straight. You fiddled desperately with the door lock high up until you escaped into the cold evening.

There was just enough time to get down Quay Street to get the eggs. Staunton's would shut the grocery shop by six.

'You remember Staunton's? Do you remember the gold lettering?' you ask me quickly, your hands going like the clappers.

'I do,' I lie.

'Do you remember that reeded glass on the windows?' you ask.
I nod, lie again.

Always the men sitting on polished oak stools up the shop's front, supping pints with rum chasers, their shiny suit pants threadbare, sleeves rolled up as they drank. Always smoke catching your throat.

*

Mrs Staunton remarked on the day's cold harshness when you stepped inside to the ding of the shop bell. Then she hurried you down the back of the shop, following close behind to keep an eye that the supping men didn't maw you as you passed. The speckled eggs were sat on straw and you usually helped yourself. But today was different. Mrs Staunton placed the eggs into the blue carton for you, your hands still shaking.

'I pity Mrs Faye's shop girls,' Mrs Staunton said, carrying the tray back up to the front of the shop to ring them up on the till.

'I don't suppose you'd have anything going here Mrs Staunton?' you said, quickly, your bravery up with your blood. There were few shop positions in town for girls who left school early and Mrs Staunton knew this. She felt sorry for the girls about the town. She had managed her grocery alone since her Mr Staunton died in the river. She couldn't afford to take on help.

'Oh love, I'm sorry but I can't afford an extra pair of hands, much as I could do with them. There's no profit in eggs and Guinness, not as much as in fancy cakes and coffee in any case.'

You paid and thanked her quietly, trying to resist rubbing your hand off the side of your face as you backed out of the shop, bottom first, eggs last.

'Are you sure you're alright?' Mrs Staunton called out after you, but you didn't dare turn back and unbalance the eggs.

Outside, the wind cut you and instead of turning right to walk home, you turned left. The water down by the Spanish

Arch had a current that you followed in a hurry. You rushed to the water. It was terrifying but exhilarating and then, like all things you tended to rush to, you felt daft when you got there. Not knowing what to do. Unused to spectating scenery, like some people do. The fishing boats bobbed on the water and the lights were on in some of the house windows on the Long Walk. The island women were finishing up selling their fish and stood about chatting quietly in a language you understood but didn't speak. They wore their hair split down the middle and parted, pulled into a bun at the nape of their necks. The younger women had their hair braided and were not seen with the indignity of an apron. This would change over the years as necessity outweighed vanity. Small children weaved through their legs and made hide-outs in their aprons, jumping the empty baskets scattered about the grass. Some scaly mackerel lay lifeless on the bottom of the wicker baskets alongside shiny mussels.

In the river water you watched salmon slip through the hatch. As busy as women, you thought, sat on the grass, your feet pushed out ahead of you. It was nice to have shoes even if they were brown ones the colour of bathroom grout and not wine ones like Mary Quin's. It was no longer exciting to be done with school and, in turn, done with Mary Quin. The promise of freedom faded with each long day stood in the bakery. Perhaps it was better to get a slap from a teacher than a boss, but it was late to be deciding on which misfortune was worse now that you didn't sidle in beside Mary Quin on the small desk anymore. Mary Quin who fell asleep in class when her breasts started to swell and you put her hair in the inkwell for a laugh. You made the best of your forced proximity and once swore you would go swimming in the summer out to Ladies' Beach in fancy costumes, maybe lie on the sand on two large towels. You'd make up for sticking her hair in the inkwell and buy her an ice cream even though she protested about the calories, and said often that she was reducing. For some months after you finished up school, she'd stand at the window front of Faye's and stare at the cakes. It was startling how quickly she became a stranger. Once, she came into the shop front. You were in the kitchen when she ordered a large coffee cake and you so desperately wanted to go out and say hello, but she ran out of the shop just as Mrs Faye was elaborately tying ribbons around the white box.

'Silly little bitch,' Mrs Faye said, cutting her finger.

*

There came a time that you did not remember scissors can cut fingers or remember the word for your slippers. You did not remember the names of your children. You could not be left alone in the loo. You could not go outside without a sun hat and a chaperone. Soon, you could not go anywhere without a chaperone. You made an angry bald spot on your scalp from plucking grey hairs near the thinning skin on your right temple. They called this self-harm. You liked to touch your eyeball with your finger. I pulled down your hands subconsciously to distract you. This often made you worse. You stopped playing bingo. Stopped brushing your hair. You stopped singing along with songs on the radio. You had no interest in the company of other women. You stopped partaking in cookery classes, because the ovens made you cry. But the women in the dining room never tired of you like I did. They brought you gifts of jelly fruits in an assortment of colours right up to your very last moments. Sometimes they'd wait by you as they dissected them and fed them to you like mother birds.

*

Down by the river was freezing and stars were coming through the black canvas. You enjoyed the cold. It wasn't swimming season – the Atlantic sea water is dangerously cold in spring – besides, you couldn't swim in your blouse. That night, swimming was the only thing you really wanted to do, but the water was gushing and it was dark and mad. A man walked by, stopped by the railings, and stood awhile singing a song about a boat and a ferret. Your brothers had a thing for killing ferrets. Although maybe the song was about a ferry. He sang from a hole in his beard, stained tobacco-yellow.

You stared at him. You had developed a habit of staring when you were young and you never grew out of it. The eggs were clumsy and loose about the carton. The island women greeted the last of their customers as they walked away with the mackerel and mussels wrapped in newspaper. Now they were louder; laughing and thrusting their empty fish baskets about like hoopla. One spun her basket so fast it caught in the gentle breeze and turned on its side to the sea.

And she howled as if all the world's fish were rolling down the side of the bank.

The basket made its way to the gushing sea and you jumped up and rushed to it, unsettling the eggs in the grass beside you as you hurried, and running to the water, you remembered your shoes, caught a grip of yourself, considered what would happen to you if they got wet. So, changing course, you side-stepped down the side of the bank and grabbed the basket with your two hands. It stank, and iridescent scales flashed in its hardened reeds. You walked back up along the wild grass, heart beating. The woman had her hand over her mouth. The man had stopped his song about ferrets. You returned the basket. She just nodded. The singer started up again.

It had been stupid to come here.

It had been crazy to think about swimming so late in the evening, to want to wash the heat out of your face, that unbridled fucking aftershock which comes after surges of adrenaline. All the giddy plans of leaving Mrs Faye had disappeared. School would never have you back. You'd have to repeat the year with your younger brothers, the twins. Mrs Staunton had had her chance to offer you something. Even just down the back packing the hen eggs or filling flour. The blood was hot in your ears. Your breasts were a stupid trespass and the shoes on your feet were suddenly girlish.

And the eggs were cracked.

The cardboard was soaking in the wobbly albumen, one of the yolks still intact and bobbing in the broken shell, surviving momentarily, until you stuck your finger into it. Then you sucked it, before sitting back down to watch the currents take the women home in the currachs, back to the island to fill baskets for tomorrow.

And you waited in town so late that the pubs closed and you watched the men fall out of Staunton's and Mrs Staunton lifted the big wooden slats over the windows and pulled a shawl tight around her, and on the streets, drunks rattled out songs of love and loss, tales of men who'd fought and died, and great bellowing songs of someone's bravery as they slipped roughshod under the street lamps, weaving about in circles, before determining a straight line was the only way home.

At home you took your punishment from the woman in the scullery who had waited up to slap the other cheek, hard, for the children gone to bed with their bellies bet on their backs.

*

We left the ice cream melting in its bowl in the dining hall and you went back to your room.

'I'll swim now,' you said, fussing about the bed. 'Before it's too late.'

'Ok,' I said.

And you went into the bathroom and stood underneath the shower and I turned it on for you, without undressing you, and placed towels all about the floor. You stood under the water for the longest time, your blouse soaked through.

'It's time to come out now,' I said, after some time had passed.

'No, no, I can do this ...' you called out. 'I can do this forever. It never stops coming, water.'

'I see,' I said. 'I bet you can. Are you swimming?'

'I am,' you said. 'Do you have the wine for Mrs Faye?'

'I do.'

'Great,' you said.

I lifted a towel and went to you and you looked at it and turned angry as I began to remove your clothes to dry you, starting with your feet.

'We used to have bits of linoleum tiles in our shoes, you know, to stop the rain from getting in,' you said, holding the top of my head with your hands.

'Did you?'

'Yes. Now pour her a glass,' you said. 'Quickly.'

'I already have,' I said, rubbing the towel up along your rice paper skin, the scaly shins, silvery threads, the purple bluish veins.

Sitting on the bed I patted dry your ringlets.

'Red, I hope,' you said. Always red for Mrs Faye. 'I can't wait to tell her I've been swimming in the mad ocean and that I was so happy. It'll kill her.'

Our Dear Ladies Have Outnumbered Us

Jan Carson

Angelica moves in on a Wednesday.

We are out for a walk when she arrives. Every morning between *Loose Women* and lunch, we take our dear ladies for a walk. We walk in a different direction each day. There are only two directions available.

Turning left leads to the People's Park. Our ladies like to stare at the children playing on the swings. The parents don't mind so long as they keep their distance. They are not so understanding when our ladies shout or grab; recently there have been a number of incidents. There is also a duck pond in the park. Ducks are more predictable than children. We try to steer our ladies towards the ducks, though we only feed them on Monday mornings. It is something of a palaver, ensuring our ladies do not eat the bread themselves. Molly and Dot are at the stage where everything they're given – from hand soap to stale pan loaf – goes directly into their mouths.

A right turn takes us down High Street to the newsagent on the corner. Our ladies prefer the High Street route. They enjoy peeking into shop windows and saying hello to the people we pass. At the gates they veer naturally towards the right and, on left-turning days, have to be steered in the opposite direction. They are like a flock of stubborn sheep. We give our ladies money to spend in the newsagent. A pound for sweeties. A little more for a magazine, though we can't stretch to the glossies. The top shelf stuff is strictly forbidden. It makes our ladies too excitable. We let them make their own selections. It's important to preserve a sense of independence. Obviously, we supervise. Most days they pick the same bar of chocolate or packet of sweets. They are drawn to those with colourful wrappers. Margaret likes an ice pop, even in winter. Dot always nicks a packet of cheesy Wotsits. Frisking her before leaving has become part of our routine.

We turn left on Mondays, Wednesdays and Fridays; right, on alternate days. Sunday is Visitors' Day. It is up to each friend and family member to decide whether they take their lady out for a stroll, sit in the garden or in the common room. Those wishing to walk must fill in the appropriate form. We aren't required to fill in forms. We can take our ladies out whenever we like.

We are not expecting Angelica this early. She's down to arrive later this evening, just before *Coronation Street*. To be honest, we aren't expecting Angelica at all. In her notes, she's down as 'Angela – *goes by Angie*.' Of course, we don't mind calling her whatever she wants. We have completed the special training. There's no point arguing with a lady who's got a notion in her head. It's easier just to play along.

When we return from our walk, Angelica's already installed in the kitchen. She's working her way through a bowl of soup and a hunk of crusty bread. It's always soup for lunch on Wednesdays. We prepare three different kinds: cream of tomato, chicken broth and a special packet one – sometimes onion, sometimes mushroom – for Frances, who is coeliac. We don't mind making different soups if it keeps our ladies happy. It's just a matter of opening tins.

Angelica's not like our other ladies. She is wearing lipstick at the table. It's the same bright shade as a post box; an ever so slightly redder red than the tomato soup now coating her lips. She is also boldly dressed. She wears high heels, plastic beads and a furry, leopard-print coat. None of our ladies bother with makeup anymore. On Sundays they occasionally ask for a frock. Mostly they just wear jogging bottoms around the place; cardigans, slippers and pale baggy sweaters; whatever is most comfortable. We label their clothes with indelible marker, but all their clothes look similar. Occasionally items get mixed up. Mostly jumpers and cardigans. We've never had a fancy lady like Angelica before. Our other ladies are fascinated. They are not subtle. They stare and stare.

'Who are you?' asks Sandra. (Sandra is usually the first to speak.)

'Who is she?' echoes Frances. (Frances and Sandra are best friends.)

Kathleen slides in behind Angelica's chair. She strokes the fake fur collar on her coat. As her hand moves backwards and forwards rhythmically, she emits the same soft, almost feline hum she makes when the therapy dog comes to visit and she gets to nurse him on her lap.

'That's my bowl,' announces Dot. It isn't really anyone's bowl. Angelica's not to know this. She has only just arrived.

While everyone groups around the table, noising and fussing noisily, Molly swipes a hunk of bread and a salt cellar. She slips both into her cardigan pockets, bread in the left, salt in the right. We notice. It's our job to notice small infringements of the rules. We'll make sure they don't leave the kitchen. We're always finding Molly's swag secreted about the place. Inanimate objects aren't so bad; hard, solid items like coins, mugs or remotes. Food is different. Food squishes and sours and leaves a stain. It must be found and binned before it goes off.

Sandra and Frances sit down opposite Angelica. They place their hands on the table, palms down, and glare. 'Talk,' says Sandra, 'tell us everything. Who the bloody hell are you?' She repeats this phrase in perfect Spanish. Sandra used to live in Spain. In stressful moments she is prone to translate herself. Frances makes her hand into a fist. She bangs it against the tabletop. *Chhrrumpph. Chhrrumpph. Chhrrumpph.* Her papery flesh sounds like a buttered scone making contact with the wood. Frances and Sandra watch a lot of crime programmes: *Father Brown Investigates, Midsomer Murders, A Touch of Frost.* They're partial to a murder in the afternoon. There doesn't seem to be any harm in this. Sometimes they pretend to be TV cops. They're interrogating Angela now; playing good cop and bad cop, though it's hard to tell which is which. They pull the same schtick with us when demanding an extra chocolate biscuit or a DVD on Saturday night. Angelica doesn't appear intimidated. Perhaps she's used to being interrogated. Perhaps she's just oblivious.

'Hi,' she says, 'it's really nice to meet you all. Sorry, I started without you. I just love …' She pauses and glances down at her bowl as if waiting for the contents to introduce themselves. It's a look we recognise. Our ladies are always misplacing words. We know not to rush Angelica. We give her time to find the word for soup or something similarly hot and wet. It takes a few seconds before she speaks. 'I just love this kind of thing,' she says. 'I'm sorry, I couldn't resist.' She grins at the ladies; a big red, soupy lipstick grin. 'You can call me Angelica,' she says.

Molly repeats the word '*Angelica*' over and over, rumbling it round her mouth like a sucky sweet. Sandra asks if she's a film star or a person off the telly. As she says this, she swoops her arm round in a slow, wide arc taking in all of Angelica: the lipstick, the clothes, the perfectly bobbed hair. 'She might be one of those women who wears clothes in magazines,' Frances suggests. Dot is mumbling to herself, 'That's my bowl. She took my bowl.'

Angelica seems pleased to be the centre of attention. She lifts her water glass and toasts the table. 'To new friends,' she says. Some of our ladies lift a glass or teacup in response. Molly raises the margarine tub. Sandra simply lifts her hand again and waves across the table, slowly, regally, like the Queen. One by one and all at once, our ladies fall for Angelica. It happens so quickly. In a heartbeat. In a rush. One minute they are our own dear ladies: sweet, familiar and dependent. The next they're under Angelica's spell. We don't yet understand what this means.

We have six ladies in residence. There are also six of us on rotation: two on nights, when it's quieter; three through the day. There's a pleasing symmetry to this arrangement. We are, in total, a round dozen, perfectly balanced like a see-saw or a set of old-fashioned baking scales. This new addition upsets the balance. Now our dear ladies outnumber us. Seven to six. Thirteen in total. Thirteen's a number we'd prefer to avoid. To accommodate Angelica, we move Frances into Sandra's room. Neither woman thinks to complain. They spend every waking moment together. They are delighted to be roomies now. Sandra insists they're off to Guide Camp. Frances is back in boarding school. 'Yes,' we say, 'what fun you'll have.' We remind them that it's lights out at ten. No chit chatting in the dark. It is easier just to play along.

There is no question of Angelica sharing a room. She's brought three large suitcases of clothes and at least two dozen pairs of shoes. She requires a wardrobe of her own and, according to her notes, is used to having plenty of space. Until yesterday she had her own bungalow. There's a blank white space for '*next of kin*'. No children. No husband. No relatives. In the '*other comments*' section, someone's written, '*no contact with partner since diagnosis*', and in brackets, next to this, the word '*bastard*'. We presume the partner was a man. On paper there's little difference between Angelica and our other ladies aside from this distinct lack of friends or family.

We only take ladies who've been recently diagnosed. They're all still capable of the basics: feeding, washing, toileting. Some stay with us for a couple of months. Others, like Frances, have been here for years. It is impossible to say how long each will take to deteriorate. Friends and families often press us to put a number on it. Two months. Six months. A year. Three years. They want to calculate the cost. It's pricey enough, living here. 'Depends,' we say. Or sometimes, if they've asked one time too often: 'How long's a piece of string?' We deliver this pronouncement with a slight note of exasperation, a shrug and a noticeable tightening of the lips.

When our ladies become too difficult, we transfer them to 'the Other Place'. They're all aware of this arrangement. We explain it carefully before they move in here. It is possible – probable even – that each lady imagines she will be impervious, sharp enough to beat this thing which we never mention by name or even allude to. It's not dementia, nor even the d-word. It isn't doting or going downhill. It is simply an unspoken word. It hangs, immediate as the roof, over every second of our days. We've never had a lady who managed to beat it, though sometimes one will die of something else before requiring a transfer to the Other Place.

Angelica's likely to be here for some time. She has young-onset: she's only just celebrated her sixtieth. According to the GP notes, she has mild confusion, mild aphasia and mild delusions. We are not fooled by this GP or his notes. There's nothing mild about Angelica. She's a tiny hurricane. It takes her less than twenty-four hours to turn the whole place upside down.

It begins at breakfast. Our ladies usually appear around eight in their dressing gowns and sleeping gear. This morning they are notably late. The table is set; place mats squashed up to make room for Angelica. The orange juice is already poured. Pills decanted into tiny plastic cups. Cereal boxes arranged in the centre of the table. 'Like skyscrapers,' Kathleen says. Every morning. As if she's only just thought of it. The toast has been toasted in anticipation of our ladies' imminent arrival. It lies sodden on the big toast plate. It's almost half past eight before the first of them appears.

Frances and Sandra come in together. They are wearing their Sunday visitor frocks, accessorised with every item of jewellery they own. They've tried to apply makeup. It has not been a great success. Molly appears a few minutes later. She is wearing her own creation: a kind of toga, fashioned from bedsheets, worn off the shoulder to reveal an inch of greying bra strap and a generous portion of pale, chicken flesh. Kathleen has done 'something' to her hair. Margaret appears in her dressing gown, to which she's attached a cape with safety pins. On closer inspection the cape turns out to be the good velvet curtains from the common room. Only Dot looks like she routinely looks.

When Angelica arrives, immaculate in a pink trouser suit, she helps herself to a bowl of Special K before addressing the other ladies. 'Well,' she says, 'don't we all look gorgeous today?' Our ladies light up like glow-worms. 'Do you really think so?' Sandra asks, and we play along. 'Absolutely gorgeous,' we say.

We make our ladies change for their walk. It is easy enough to convince them. Outside's no place for fancy clothes. It could rain. There might be mud. 'Birds will poo on us from heaven,' suggests Molly. Molly's a little obsessed with birds. She once brought a dead pigeon home from the park and kept it for weeks in her sock drawer. 'Exactly,' we agree, 'there could be birds.' We cajole them into their regular coats. Today is a Thursday. We have every intention of turning right. Our ladies know this. At the gates they veer instinctively towards the High Street and the possibility of sweets.

Angelica does not follow. Angelica leads. She doesn't turn right or even left. She checks for traffic, then strides wilfully across the road.

'I'm late,' she cries.

'Late for what?' we holler back.

'For ...' she searches for the lost word, glancing up at down the pavement at the lampposts and kerbstones. 'I'm late,' she eventually says, 'for the thing I do every day. You know ... the thing ... in the place.'

'Work?' suggests Margaret.

'Yes, that's it. I'm late for work,' Angelica replies.

And just like that, all our ladies forget the newsagent and the High Street. Every one of them's late for work. Work is one of those stretchy words. It shapes itself differently for each of them. Work is a hospital to Molly and Dot, and a high-windowed classroom for Kathleen. Frances pictures a desk and typewriter. Sandra and Margaret are stay-at-home types. They're rushing home to tackle the laundry and the grocery list. There is no turning them. Our ladies believe themselves late for work and it's easier just to play along.

We follow them as they follow Angelica, across the road and down a side street, through a warren of alleys and lanes, over the supermarket car park, to the graveyard on the edge of town, where Angelica stops abruptly. She has a very particular look on her face. We are all familiar with this look. It is the look of a person who's just woken up in an unfamiliar room. She stares at the headstones, attempting to orientate herself. She reads out the words on the cemetery sign. The name. The instructions for visitors. The opening hours.

'It's a dead place,' she says, 'why did you bring us to a dead place?'

'Dead place,' says Dot, and points at the graveyard.

'I know somebody who died,' says Margaret. 'A man. Jim. My man. Is Jim dead?'

'Jim's dead,' says Kathleen with tremendous certainty.

Frances and Sandra begin to weep.

Margaret's quick to harmonise.

While the other ladies stand there howling, Molly stoops down stealthily and swipes an angel ornament off some poor woman's plot. It's not the first time we've faced a situation like this. Hysteria spreads quickly amongst our ladies. Last December, when we let them watch *The Muppet Christmas Carol* we were, for many weeks after, plagued by ladies seeing ghosts. It's best to swoop in and distract quickly before proper panic can take hold.

'Well,' we say, with some bravado, 'that's work over for another day. We should probably be heading home.'

We watch our ladies carefully. We can see they are conflicted. They look at us with big, sad eyes. Then they turn to look at the graveyard. Then they glance at Angelica, who waits a second, and another second, before she decides to cooperate. It isn't her decision to make. We're manipulating our ladies, sweeping them up in a grand subterfuge. And yet, there's something defiant in the way she words herself. 'Yes,' she agrees, 'it's time we got home and put the dinner on.' It's as if she knows we know she's just playing along.

We are only in the door – still removing coats and outdoor shoes – when Molly starts moaning, 'I'm hungry starving. Can we eat?'

'Is it breakfast now?' asks Margaret.

We correct her gently. It's dinner time. Thursday dinner's a favourite with our ladies: fish fingers, spuds and peas.

'No, no,' insists Margaret, 'it's definitely breakfast time.'

Perhaps we are imagining this, but for a brief and fleeting second, Angelica's lips appear to move involuntarily. It could be they're forming two distinct syllables – break and fast – but the light isn't great in the hall. It could just as easily be a smile she's trying to suppress. No sound is made yet Molly's somehow got a hold of the word. 'Breakfast,' she mumbles, 'breakfast, fastbreak, break the fast.' She does a little stompy dance, tapping her socked toes against the linoleum.

The idea is contagious. Soon, all our ladies are demanding breakfast. They want soldier toast and boiled eggs, Rice Krispies with sugar and milky tea. It has just gone five. It isn't breakfast time for hours, but what's the harm in swapping one meal for another? 'Well,' we say, 'it could be fun.' Something to raise our ladies' spirits after the incident in the cemetery. We'll have breakfast for dinner, just this once. Our ladies are nonplussed. The novelty is wasted on them. It is morning in their heads. They've already bought into the pretence.

'It's breakfast time,' announces Frances. 'We should be in our jammies.'

We let them put their sleeping gear on. We don't mind these kinds of distractions. Breakfast for dinner's a bit of a laugh. It's easier just to play along. They tell you, in training, it's not really lying. It's more like play-acting; the sort of thing you do with children when they imagine themselves to be monsters or puppy dogs. There isn't any harm in it, at least that's what we've been telling ourselves. Then the witchy woman arrives.

Angelica's the first to see her. She's standing by the common room window, peering out into the dark garden beyond. We haven't had time to rehang the curtains. They're lying in a heap on Margaret's bed. The rest of our ladies are watching telly – a programme about young couples buying holiday homes – when Angelica screams. It's not the kind of scream you hear in scary movies. It's more like the noise you make when you stub a toe. High-pitched. Insistent. Elemental. We turn to find Angelica, horrored and pointing out the window, her finger resting lightly against the glass.

'There's a woman ... a witchy woman, looking in,' she says.

This isn't the first time there's been confusion about reflections. Our ladies frequently see things in puddles and shop windows. Bathroom mirrors are a bloody nightmare. We should explain this phenomenon to Angelica, simply like you'd tell a child. *There's no witchy woman, my love. You're just seeing your own reflection in the glass.* But Frances is demanding a hot-water bottle and Molly's trying to thieve Sandra's watch and wee Margaret is making the face she makes when she desperately needs the loo. There's a lot going on this evening. It is easier just to play along. 'Don't worry,' we say, 'the witchy woman can't get in. We'll go outside in a second and chase her away.' Later we'll wish we'd taken a different tack.

Our ladies are slow to bed tonight and it's eleven before we get round to doing the evening checks. All the bedroom lights are out. The whole building's quiet. It normally is at this time of night. Most of our ladies take a mild sedative and sleep peacefully until seven or eight.

We begin our checks at one end of the corridor, opening doors quietly, peeking inside. At first, we are shocked. By the third room, we're expecting it. Our ladies aren't sleeping. They're sitting bolt upright in their beds, wide-eyed and staring at the opposite wall. When we try to coerce them into a sleeping position, they make no sound, not even a murmur. Their eyes are open, but they don't respond to our gentle questions. *Are you ok, my love? Did you have a bad dream?* Their arms and legs are stiffer than usual, like the arms and legs of baby dolls. We would not describe this state as a trance. It is more of a waking dream. We've read about similar phenomena but never seen a case in real life.

Only Dot is sleeping normally.

When we check on Angelica, she's sitting up like the other ladies. She's unresponsive when we talk to her. But her eyes are different. They're sharp and quick. There's a light behind them; a clever light. She blinks when we manoeuvre her on to her side, blinks again when we tuck her in.

We write everything down in the incident book and continue our checks throughout the night, calling in at half-hour intervals. In the morning our ladies seem fine.

We have breakfast for breakfast. All our ladies appear at the normal time. They are dressed in regular breakfast clothes. Even

Angelica is wearing pyjamas: a striking silk pair in opal green, heavily embroidered, with a matching robe. Kathleen sits next to her, casually stroking her sleeve. 'You're all green,' she says, 'like a big elevator.' 'Alligator,' snaps Sandra and automatically translates herself. '*Caimán.*' She's grumpy this morning. She gets like this when she's underslept. We make no mention of what happened last night. We don't know how to speak of it. Instead, we grin and say, 'Breakfast again. Two meals in a row. That's a bit mad, isn't it?' Our ladies stare at us like we're the mad ones. No one remembers what they ate last night.

Breakfast proceeds without incident. There's the normal nonsense chatter. The normal demands for more runny jam and chocolate spread. We leave our ladies sitting at the table to make a start on the breakfast dishes. We're standing at the sink when a pointed silence descends upon the room. It is not a gradual quiet. It comes down like a garage door. One second there's a companionable hum. The next an utter absence of sound. We turn to see our ladies frozen at the table, mouths hung open, thin necks strained. Their eyes are bugging out behind prescription lenses and cataracts as they stare at the skylight above their heads. Margaret is the first to speak. 'The witchy woman's up there,' she says, raising her hand to claw at the air. All the women nod in agreement. It's impossible to tell who started this.

Only Dot is unconcerned. She's pulling the crusts off a slice of toast. She has her eyes trained on Angelica, though this may be a coincidence. Dot's always been drawn to bright colours and Angelica, in her silk pyjamas, is the brightest thing in the room.

God forgive us, we haven't the sense to see what's coming. We smile at our ladies and play along. We do not tell them it's a delusion. There's no witchy woman looking in. We don't want our ladies to know their brains are playing tricks. Such a realisation might frighten them. It seems more sensible to make a game of it.

A delegation's dispatched to the garden, ready to shoo the witchy women away. Harsh words are spoken, loudly for the benefit of our ladies who are watching on through the kitchen window. Kathleen says we should shoot the witchy woman with a gun. We have no gun, but as a kind of compromise, several large pinecones are pitched on to the roof, haphazardly and with exaggerated vitriol. A cheer goes up from inside. Afterwards we insist the witchy woman won't be coming back. We claim to have seen her fly away on a broomstick. She said she didn't like it here.

For a few hours our ladies are fine. Sandra and Frances watch some telly in the common room. Dot and Kathleen work on a jigsaw. Molly steals pieces at intervals. Margaret and Angelica sit together at the kitchen table doing mindful colouring in. The witchy woman does not return until we're out for our morning walk.

It's a Friday; a left-turning day. There are no complaints from our ladies when we shuffle them down to the park. It is clear and bright, a great day for being outside. The witchy woman is outside too. She's waiting for our ladies, floating just beneath the duck pond's surface. Kathleen spots her. Kathleen screams. She pitches an empty can of Fanta into the pond. Our ladies rush to her assistance. 'Kill the witchy woman,' shouts Margaret. Sandra removes one of her walking shoes and tries to throw it into the water. After this, it's a free for all.

Our ladies rifle through the rubbish bins for cans and other missiles to chuck. Molly, seeing an opportunity, pockets several empty cigarette packets before they can be thrown into the pond. Frances pelts handful after handful of gravel and soil. Dot wanders off to sit on a bench. Dot doesn't do well with noise or fuss. Our ladies soon draw the park-keeper's attention. He is irate. We are setting a bad example for children, throwing rubbish into the pond. Frances tries to tell him there's a witchy woman in the water. It comes out Spanish. The park-keeper doesn't understand. Sandra tries to explain in English. It all sounds a bit mad. We are politely asked to leave.

On the way home, Margaret spots the witchy woman in a puddle. Sandra sees her trapped behind the window of the podiatrist where she gets her corns seen too. Frances spies her in the back seat of a passing Renault Megane. Back home, Molly locks herself in her ensuite bathroom for an hour. She whispers to us through the door, 'The witchy woman's in my sink. Don't worry. I'm going to put water on her until she's dead.' We can hear both taps going full blast. By the time we find the master key, the water's running under the door. The bedroom carpet's sodden. It will probably need replaced.

Angelica never sees the witchy woman again herself, but she's almost always next to the lady who does. After the second or third glimpse, we begin to notice a recurring pattern. Angelica appears in the common room. Angelica pops her head into someone's room. She sidles up to another lady. She sits next to her on the sofa. She passes her a cup of tea. A few seconds later, the shout goes up; *The witchy woman's back again!* As soon as the news has broken, Angelica starts screaming along with the rest of them. There's a kind of mask which slips across her face. Her forehead creases along set lines. Her lips retract into themselves. Her eyes grow small and vital as buttonholes. She is not so much shocked as playing the part of a lady who's shocked and horrified.

We ask her to step into the garden, just for a few minutes, for a wee chat. 'Nothing to worry about,' we say. We sit together on the bench next to the big rhododendron bush. We ask Angelica about the witchy woman. We assure her we won't be angry. We never get angry with our ladies even when they drop their tea mugs on the floor, or rip the wallpaper, or wet the bed. We don't get angry, but we do keep note. Too many incidents of this nature and we transfer them to the Other Place.

'The witchy woman, she's not real, is she?' we ask. We use our kindest voices. We pat Angelica on the knee. There are certain parts of old ladies which are safe to touch in a friendly manner: knees, shoulders, elbows and hands. The parts in the middle are to be avoided. We've all done the course on safeguarding. We know how to protect ourselves. Angelica doesn't respond. She is silent and also stiff.

'It has to stop,' we continue, using a slightly firmer voice. 'All this nonsense about witchy women, it has to stop right now,' we say. 'The other ladies are terrified. Do you hear us Angelica, love? It really, really has to stop.'

But Angelica isn't listening. She's gone a funny colour of white; off white, really, like the colour of cornflour. She raises an immaculately manicured finger and points at the common room window. She makes a kind of strangled sound, as if there's something solid stuck in her throat, struggling to move up or down.

'What is it, Angelica?' we say.

'The thing ... the bad thing with the face,' she rasps, 'the woman thing is inside now.'

We stare at the common room window. Dot is standing there. She's shoved her face up against the glass. Her nose is squidged. Her mouth is gaping and cavernous. She does this sometimes, for a laugh. We've asked her not to. Her slabbers leave unsightly marks. She tends to ignore us. She likes the way the cold glass feels. 'That's not the witchy woman,' we say. 'That's just Dot doing her fish impression.' Angelica doesn't respond. She levers herself up off the bench and walks away.

All day we wonder if we've made a mistake. Perhaps we should look into transferring Angelica. Everything's felt unbalanced since she arrived. We decide not to take our ladies for a walk. It feels safer just to stay inside. At the usual walking time, Dot puts her coat on and stands at the door. We tell her it's raining, it's far too wet to go outside. She doesn't even question the lie. 'Oh, yes,' she says, 'a big storm, I think, is on the way.'

None of our other ladies notice we haven't been for a walk today. They are more docile than usual; no doubt tired from losing sleep. Several of them take an afternoon nap. We wake them in time for dinner. It's a chippy tea on Saturdays; our ladies' favourite meal of the week. The witchy woman doesn't join us. There's been no mention of her since our chat in the garden. Maybe Angelica's got the message and we've seen the last of her. Everybody's in better form. We watch *Strictly* together in the common room. All our ladies are down and settled by ten to ten. We like them to have a good night's sleep on Saturdays. Visitors' Day the following day can be exhausting. They need all the energy they can get.

We do not hear our dear ladies leaving. They are very quiet when they go.

We check them at ten and don't check again till almost one. It's impossible to know how long they've been outside. We're sprawled out on the common room sofa. Shoes kicked off. Slippers on. The TV's blaring. The curtains – recently rehung – are drawn. It's just a regular Saturday evening. We always watch a movie on Saturday. Obviously, we don't drink on duty but sometimes we order a pizza in. We make a kind of night of it. We're watching *Pretty Woman* – we're big fans of Julia Roberts. She's so pretty but she's not one bit up herself – when we hear a scream outside. We know without looking that it's Dot. Dot's from Scotland originally. You can hear her accent when she coughs or laughs. She even sounds Scottish when she screams.

There's a frantic scramble for outdoor shoes. We are tripping over each other trying to get out the door. A mug of tea's upended in the furore. By the time we get round to mopping it up, it will have left a permanent stain. All our ladies are on the lawn, gathered in front of the sycamore tree. They're barefoot in their nighties and pyjamas. They're making an awful humming noise; low and demented like a fridge that's about to give up the ghost. They've formed a loose circle. Dot's in the centre of the circle, sat on the grass with her nightdress drawn over her knees. She has her arms roofed above her head. She screams, draws breath and screams again, as the other ladies pitch pinecones viciously at her head.

We run frantically across the lawn. We shout all the things you'd expect us to shout: 'Stop it' and 'What's going on?'; 'Holy shit' and 'Bloody hell'. Our ladies pause. They freeze with their arms by their sides. They do not turn or look at us. Their eyes are cloudy and faraway. Like the eyes of hard drinking men. When we ask, 'What on earth is going on?' their gaze drifts towards Angelica, then suddenly darts away.

We take them inside. We put them to bed. We ask them individually and collectively, 'What on earth were you doing throwing pinecones at poor Dot?' Molly and Margaret insist they weren't. Kathleen says she doesn't know anybody called Dot. Sandra says, 'That's what you do with witchy women.' Frances is quick to agree. 'Remember, you showed us,' she says, 'you have to throw pinecones at the witchy woman, if you want her to go away.'

Angelica says nothing. We watch while she slarries her face in night cream and climbs into bed. 'Night,' she says like it's just an ordinary bedtime. It looks as if she's smiling smugly in her sleep though this might just be how her mouth looks when she's dreaming.

We have to give Dot a stronger sedative. We have to sit with her until she drifts off.

Once our ladies are down and settled, we regroup in the common room. Something must be done about Angelica. In the morning we'll contact the Other Place and ask if she can be transferred. 'Immediately,' we'll say, 'this morning ideally, or this afternoon.' We are not sure how we'll convince them to take her away. It's not as if she's deteriorated. She's only been with us for four days. We want to say Angelica is corrupting our ladies but it doesn't sound sensible when we say it. It sounds like something we've made up. We finish the movie. We make more tea. We decide upon the party line. Angelica must leave because she has upset the balance. We can manage six ladies but seven has proven a bit overwhelming. This sounds almost believable.

In the morning Dot is gone.

Our ladies are silent on the subject. They appear for breakfast at the usual time. They listen to the service on the wireless, as is their custom on Sunday mornings. Afterwards, in anticipation of visitors, they change into their favourite frocks.

When we ask our ladies where Dot's gone, they look at us blankly as if Dot's not a word they recognise.

'Dot. Dot. Dot,' says Molly, tapping her index finger against the wall.

We threaten to get the police involved.

'*Policía*,' says Sandra. Frances instinctively takes her hand.

Angelica shrugs and emits a peevish, teenage sigh, as if to say, why are you bothering me with this nonsense?

'Honestly,' we say, 'this isn't a game. We really will have to call the police.'

Our ladies are unmoved by this threat. There are once again six of us and six of them but this no longer feels like a balanced set up. Our dear ladies have outnumbered us.

Heatwave

Oona Frawley

It was midsummer, towards the peak of the heatwave, when the call came about Pat. Maura and Ellie were in the back garden repainting the shed and sketching plans for a mural on the concrete wall that divided them from their neighbours. Maura tried to keep her niece occupied, giving her holidays structure day to day, though sometimes this demanded too much of her. Ellie, fifteen and sharp as her own collarbones, watched jewels of sweat magnify Maura's freckles and knew that it was too much for her aunt. She was old enough to entertain herself – she had two Stephen King novels upstairs, borrowed from the library, and would have been glad to lie in the sun reading – but Maura kept elaborating on the mural plans until the dirty white wall was covered in annotations and shapes. When Ellie looked at it, she thought of a programme she'd seen on the expansion of the universe, scientific formulae and numbers appearing rapidly across a massive board as the researcher spoke. In all likeliness the rain would return before the mural was finished, but Ellie didn't say so. You could say something like that to your mother but not your aunt.

When the phone rang, Maura went in with relief, glad of an excuse to step out of the sun. Ellie saw her through the glass, taking the receiver off the hook and then perching on a stool she kept nearby, dabbing her forehead with a tea towel. She continued painting the warm slats of the shed, watching tiny bubbles popping as the liquid absorbed into the grey wood that was so hot and dry. They were painting it a solid sky blue, because Maura wanted something cheerful to look at in winter, with white trim round the door and the one small window for contrast. The wood seemed so parched Ellie thought it would take at least one extra coat.

After a few moments Maura returned with two glasses of blackcurrant. Her mouth was already working as if rehearsing the news she was about to deliver and Ellie, seeing this, put the brush down immediately and stood up. She relieved Maura of the glasses since her aunt's hands had begun to tremble slightly and braced herself for some news about her mother. Had she fallen? Lashed out at another resident as had happened once before? But when Maura began to speak it turned out she'd been completely off base. Ellie's Uncle Pat – Maura and Mum's brother – had leapt out of his car at a traffic light in central Paris. 'In the 14th arrondissement,' Maura added, though Ellie had never been to Paris and the detail meant nothing to her. In the car were his wife and teenagers, Ellie's cousins, en route back to Ireland after their holiday.

Back in the doldrums of bleak February, Paris had been a hot spark in Pat's mind, an add-on to the Eurocamp experience which he'd spoken of with starry eyes. Maura wondered if the baffling networks of roads had upset Pat. She couldn't be sure for she'd heard the whole story second hand from Pat's wife. As if mid-race, he'd pegged down a winding avenue and quickly disappeared from sight. The light changed. His wife had had to drive on, shouting at the kids in the back seat to pull the wavering door to. Wasn't it strange that her impulse hadn't been to go after her husband but rather to obey traffic regulations? People's natures could be strange. This was something to think about, Maura said.

Pat's wife Anne was now in a police station. The kids were in the car outside. She'd reported Pat missing but the police told her that he was an adult with no history of mental illness, had his wallet in his pocket, and should be fine. This meant 'he wasn't really *missing*', they'd said, with exaggerated French air quotes. Were there problems in the marriage? Could he have a lover in France? They'd advised that Anne continue her travels. If Pat came to harm in Paris, he would be taken care of, but they thought, by the sound of things, he was probably able to take care of himself. Anne had whispered down the phone that the way they'd spoken to her was just humiliating. Then she'd asked Maura if she thought she should drive on. Maura had sat silently on the stool by the telephone, looking out at Ellie as her blue brush stroked the wood confidently. She'd said, yes, Anne should drive on.

Ellie, at once relieved for her mother not being in trouble and also worried for Pat, got her aunt to sit down on the bench they'd sanded and painted with wood preservative the previous Easter. It was a weird brown-green. Maura had already pointed out that it wouldn't match the blue. Ellie suspected it would become a project for another school holiday. Maura was quiet, examining her drained glass, turning it this way and that so Ellie caught exaggerated green gleams of grass through its curves. Ellie suggested Pat might have been desperate for the loo – or carsick. He had money so he'd be alright. Maura nodded her head up and down too many times. She wasn't listening to Ellie's actual words. Privately they both wondered if Pat had been suddenly overcome by the need to move and be uncontained, if he'd flown from the car accordingly. They'd both seen this before, after all. For a good while they simply sat in the heat, quiet, holding their empty glasses and thinking about Pat, somewhere in Paris.

*

The next day, Anne arrived home. An unforecast drizzle had interrupted the outdoor work, so Ellie had put the brushes in jam jars of water in the one-coat shed and baked a cake. It was plain vanilla sponge because Maura reckoned Anne and the cousins would need something simple in their tummies after a holiday in France, especially seeing they'd come home without Pat. Ellie had dusted the sponge with icing sugar. The air was so damp that by the time they arrived at Anne's the sugar had disappeared; there was only a sticky sheen on top of the cake and it looked unappetising. Anne fell into her sister-in-law's arms and cried while Ellie put the kettle on and dusted the cake with more icing sugar. When the tea was ready Anne was coaxed to sit at the table. Ellie's cousins were upstairs. She figured her presence would make whatever they were feeling worse. They'd be thinking about the state her mother had ended up in. But after a little while, the older two came down.

Kate and Colm ate the plain cake and drank mugs of instant coffee, adjusting back to Irish habits. While their mother clutched her teacup in silence, they described their father's disappearance. They were eager to share their version of events. Because they hadn't been inside the police station, this was their first opportunity to discuss the incident with anyone besides their mum. You could tell that as they spoke they were trying to make sense of what had happened, even if they were unable to. Michelle, younger than Ellie by a year, eventually appeared in the doorway, lured by the sound of her siblings' talking. Her nose and forehead, sunburnt during the Bordeaux stage of their trip, were peeling dramatically so she looked like some strange fruit, overripe and splitting its skin.

'Sit down and have some cake, love,' Maura beckoned her, but Michelle clung to the door frame.

'For God's sake, Michelle, will you come and sit down,' her mother said. 'You're making me nervous hanging on like that with your fingernails.'

'What if Dad ends up like Ellie's mum?' Michelle countered, not looking at Ellie.

'Then at least you'll know where he is,' Ellie said, and went out to wait in the car. It was locked, so she lounged against the boot, hot from the recently re-emerged sun. She stared into the deep shimmer of the metallic navy paint. There were tiny scratches from years of raising and lowering the boot for groceries, suitcases and recycling, but it was still like staring into a universe; all gleaming stars and rainbow halos.

Kate and Colm came out to apologise for their sister's behaviour.

'How is your mum anyway?' Colm asked.

'The same,' Ellie said, her palms sweating from the car's radiant heat. 'How was France?' she asked in return. 'I mean, before?'

All of their usual ease was gone. After a few minutes of forced conversation about the rest of the holiday, Ellie's cousins wondered back towards the house when her aunt appeared.

'Don't worry about Michelle,' Maura said. 'She's just rattled. You know that.'

'Yeah. They're all rattled. I get it.' Ellie waved at her retreating cousins.

'But she still shouldn't have said that about your mum.' Maura looked at Ellie directly before starting the car. 'I'm sorry, pet.' Ellie thought of Michelle's fingers on the door frame, curling around the wood, of Pat's hand on the slim handle of the car door.

'Will we stop by Mum's on the way home or do you want to wait until tomorrow?' she asked her aunt.

*

Ellie was used to newcomers and strangers mistaking her mother for a visitor, nurse or carer. Her mother strode along the gravel paths. Her walk remained purposeful and athletic.

124

Her face was smooth and her fine hair more pepper than salt. When she spotted Ellie and Maura, she beamed and continued walking, so Ellie had to fly after her and grab her arm. Her mum turned bright eyes towards her, pausing for a fractional second. Her hair sometimes flew out slightly when she stopped moving, as if she were electric when still. The strands floated like delicate cilia, silver and black, crackling with energy in the warm air.

The three of them walked for an hour, weaving about as Ellie's mum saw fit, sometimes in full laps of the garden. Sometimes they made small circles round a flowerbed, turning awkwardly together. Ellie's mum didn't acknowledge the heat, though her brow glistened and the fine hair at her temple was slick like a small child's after running. The longer they walked, the more she smiled at Ellie, now holding tight to her hand.

'She definitely knows you,' Maura said quietly. 'Look at her looking at you.'

They shared sweets that Maura produced from her handbag. Ellie's mum paused appreciatively each time Maura spiralled the wrapper to reveal another pastille. She stretched out her fine-boned hands for the sugary disk as if taking communion, some automatic memory surfacing as she waited for the sweet to be placed in her palm.

'This could go on for years,' Maura had said one night, near the beginning. Maura hadn't lied to Ellie or blurred the truth as many had encouraged her to. When her mum was diagnosed, Ellie had just turned thirteen. She'd been alive with hormones and brain networks just establishing themselves. Maura had figured the truth was best. 'Your mum's young and fit. She might remain in this state for decades. So, we need to figure a way for you and me to live with it.' Ellie loved this truth-telling in Maura. She tolerated all kinds of other things because of it, including the painting and household jobs they did together. Her aunt had taken her in, after all.

'Not many would've done it,' Ellie'd overheard a hundred times since, at school meetings, dentist appointments, even at the shops when old ladies told Maura what a good girl Ellie was to push the trolley for her.

They left when a carer came to bring Ellie's mum to tea. She waved them off blithely. Neither of them enjoyed teatimes; the ordeal of trying to get Ellie's mum to sit still for long enough to consume a meal. Maura had decided that, for Ellie's sake, they would only visit between meals, when she was at her best.

'Maybe Pat's walking,' Maura mused as they reached the car.

'Maybe,' Ellie replied. She pictured the way her mother would cry if they tried to force her to stop walking, the way her arms would turn angry, swiping and lashing like tentacles. Yes, she could easily imagine her Uncle Pat walking.

*

Ellie also loved to walk, even if this fact sometimes worried her. During summer holidays, she'd walk to the local library. She visited school friends who lived nearby and they sat on walls. They were often told to move on. Sometimes, they'd scrabble together a few pounds and walk to the Stillorgan Shopping Centre to try on clothes, then spend their money in the newsagent on salt and vinegar crisps or the cheaper ice creams. Occasionally they'd go to the cinema. But there was no money to speak of, so they mostly just sat somewhere or walked. A sixth of the country was out of work and another sixth seemed to have gone abroad; the summer roads were quiet.

When her friends weren't around and Maura didn't have anything planned, Ellie took the bus to see her mum on her own, preferring the top deck and its rattling silence. She didn't always tell Maura. She just went and walked with her mother round the gardens and paths or along the hallways if it was wet. During these visits Ellie talked to her mum differently from when Maura was present. She told her mum what was going on in her life and in her mind. Sometimes, her mum talked too, in flurries and bursts; sometimes in long, slow, fluid sentences. Her words were sculptural as cloud; soft and moving, composed of everything Ellie wanted to hear. It would be hard to explain what these exchanges meant, how deep they went into her. She could say anything. She could listen to and accept anything her mother said. Her mother seemed to feel the same.

Once, on her way out, after a conversation that had brought Ellie intense peace of mind, she'd overheard one of the carers talking about her.

'God love her,' the woman had said to a cleaner, 'she's only a child and of course she wants to spend time with her mother, but wouldn't it break your heart to see how little response she gets.'

Ellie's anger surprised her. This stranger obviously didn't know that her conversations with her mother incorporated gestures and looks which had been passing between them since she was born. When her mother blinked at Ellie and tugged her earlobe lightly it was the thousandth such motion. If her mother's elbow crooked slightly outwards from her body as Ellie fell into fast step beside her, it was because she knew her daughter would slip her arm through hers as she'd been doing since she'd grown tall enough at seven or eight. And on rare days, when Ellie's mother gathered her name from the depths of herself and crooned it aloud, Ellie's emotions would rise through her body as if a chorus of love had been sung to her. Even on the days when her mum was not at her best, Ellie was grateful simply for her presence, happy just to hold her hand. With the high scorn of a teenager, she barely acknowledged the carer again.

*

Ellie had told her mother about a boy she was drawn to. He lived round the corner from her aunt's house. She'd see him out cutting the grass for his parents and strolling with friends near the local shop. He was long and lean, newly muscled in the way that fifteen-and sixteen-year-old boys are, their bodies pushing against their clothes. All through the summer days, she'd thought about kissing him; the flick of his dark hair, how his skin would feel. A few days after Pat's disappearance as she exited the warm bus from the home – her mother's scattered conversations still singing in her ears – she'd spied him, perched alone, on a wall beside the phone box. They saw each other so often they'd begun to nod when they passed. This was an intermediate stage, Ellie thought, before kissing became a possibility; somehow people could move from greetings to conversation to kissing. She wondered how other people navigated this journey so naturally or if it was always inevitably awkward. When Ellie nodded at the boy, she was conscious of her hair feathering forward on her neck in wisps, conscious that her legs were bare and red with sunburn.

'How's it going?' she said automatically. She'd thought of the boy so often that speaking to him had somehow become instinctual.

'Alright. You?' he returned.

Ellie nodded. 'Just heading to the shop, for my aunt. No milk for the tea. The ones on the doorstep went sour with the heat.' She smiled because she was nervous.

'You live with your aunt, don't you?'

'Yeah, I do. At the Meadows.'

'Aye, I know it. I'm around at the Brook, just beyond.'

Ellie smiled. 'Well, I guess I'd better go on.'

'I can walk with you,' he said, 'if that's alright. My mate's late, dunno where he's got to.'

'I'm Ellie,' she said.

'Declan,' he replied.

When they waved goodbye at her front gate, Maura's neat navy car parked behind it, Ellie thought of telling her mother that having had a sort of conversation with this boy, she was one step closer to the kissing part.

Out back, Maura had already started on the mural. Ellie had suggested a garden scene: butterflies, birds, a tree, perhaps some bright spots of ladybirds, buttercups. But this hadn't suited Maura's vision. In the end, she'd surprised her niece by deciding on something conceptual and irregularly patterned. She was on her knees in the grass, outlining various shapes in blue: a series of green abstracts was already visible.

'I thought I'd make a start,' she said, 'seeing as it's fine.'

'No word of Pat yet?' Ellie asked, stretching out on the grass beside her.

Maura shook her head. 'Four days,' she said, not stopping her painting. 'He'd be tired walking now, wouldn't he?'

Ellie didn't reply.

'Do you ever think about what would happen to you if I did the same thing?' Maura kept a steady hand on the blue brush, awkwardly positioned near the ground.

'Sometimes,' Ellie said. 'What would happen?' The green of the grass was textured up this close, striated with light.

'I wanted to tell you. Because I knew it would be worrying you, especially now Pat's gone off on his travels.' Maura looked at her. 'I talked to Anne and Pat about it, ages ago. If you were still young, you'd go and live there. And this house would be yours when you're older … when I'm gone.'

Ellie's eyes flooded. 'The idea of you being gone!' she said. Sometimes she came close to saying the same honest things to Maura that she said to her mum. But this was as much as she could manage today with the tears imminent.

Maura nodded, touched Ellie's face and wiped her own eyes hammily to make Ellie smile. Then she laughed.

'I hope for your sake you won't have to walk the lot of us.'

*

In the end, Pat returned in a taxi. He sprung from the front seat and paused for a final few words and a laugh with the driver, then sent him off with a quick tap-tap on the car roof and a wave. By this stage Anne was out the door, a few seconds too late to have the taxi driver confirm where he'd picked Pat up.

'There were ructions,' Maura told her niece and Declan later. They were sitting side by side on the bench as Maura continued painting. 'You can imagine how Anne felt, what she said. Especially since Pat hadn't a rasher why she was so overcome. Let's just say she went from relief to fury in a trice.'

'And he's okay?' Ellie asked. Her bare leg was near Declan's and it was hard to concentrate.

'Seems to be,' Maura said, 'but I'll see for myself tomorrow. He's happy as Larry at the moment, back from his travels and not in the least concerned. Can't say where he's been or what he's been at, no receipts or anything in his pockets to give clues. Anne said it was almost as if he'd been holed up with some lover in Paris.'

Ellie was slightly mortified that Maura would mention lovers in front of Declan.

'But he hasn't been doing anything like that!' she said. 'It's Uncle Pat!'

'Ach, Ellie,' Maura smiled. 'I know he hasn't, love. But it would almost be a relief to Anne to have an explanation. I'll go and have a chat with him tomorrow when she's gone to work. Your cousins will still be asleep, no doubt. Two weeks! Where in heavens could he have been?'

The next day, after Maura had left for Pat's, Ellie worked on the mural alone. She wondered how her aunt would feel talking to him, the worry that she would try to conceal. Maybe Pat would be concerned too, now that Anne had told him what had happened. What would it be like, to have no solid recollection of what you'd done with yourself for two whole weeks? He'd probably feel more worried if he thought of

Ellie's mum. Sometimes Ellie worried about the future herself. Everyone remarked on how *young* her mother had been to get a diagnosis like that. She knew her mum's age meant some genetic connection or cause was assumed. Did her mother's condition mean that by the time Ellie was forty she'd be heading the same way? On the one hand it was ages away – she was only fifteen – on the other, it seemed not so long ago that her mum had been grand, a bit eccentric maybe, but generally grand.

Ellie was glad when Declan called round. Sitting there on the grass alone thinking about it all while she tried to paint made her sad. She missed Maura's company.

She found herself smiling as she opened the door. She was still nervous around Declan. She liked him so much. As they worked together on the mural, Ellie couldn't help thinking about the empty house. She imagined them creeping upstairs to her room, lying on her bed with the curtains drawn, the morning light exploding in lines round the edges. She managed to resist the temptation; the painting was a kind of distraction. She still didn't know how those things happened, how you went from the idea of going upstairs with someone to actually going upstairs. As they painted, Ellie told Declan about the Stephen King novel she was reading. He picked it up from the grass and read the back cover. He'd seen *The Shining*, he told her, when his older brother had rented it. It'd scared the life out of him, so he was impressed she could read the book.

Later, when they paused for lunch, he suddenly reached for her. Ellie was sitting on the grass, a plate of ham sandwiches balanced on her lap. His hand crept up her neck and into her hair. Ellie felt an unravelling in her body as their lips met. They sat on the grass, kissing. Through the soft, soft skin of his arm she felt the solidity of his skeleton. There was something reassuring and anchoring about this. When they pulled apart, they were slightly shyer, the daylight confrontational after their closed-eye kissing. Declan re-plated the sandwiches. They drank coffee on the bench in the garden, examining the mural and discussing what colours to add next.

'What happened to your mum?' Declan asked.

Ellie thought. 'She had *a little turn*,' she started. She'd rehearsed something like this so often, but her friends never really asked after her mum. Her lovely mum, who was still elementally herself, but without some totalising mechanism, the thing that pulled her all together. She didn't know how to talk to this boy, who was still essentially a stranger, even if she'd just been kissing him. 'She had a turn,' Ellie said again. 'And then things changed.' This was true. Afterwards Ellie's mum had continued to smile and chatter but she'd become a mime of herself. They were her gestures, her expressions, even some of her words, but something wasn't quite right.

'And your uncle? Did the same thing happen?'

'I don't know,' Ellie said. 'He's a bit funny.' She thought of last Christmas, when the turkey had been mostly raw and various components of the dinner scattered about the kitchen. A peeled carrot. A melon split open; one half balled. A cauldron of boiling water with a plate rattling about maniacally. But no pudding. Anne drinking wine too quickly in the conservatory because she'd been banished from the kitchen for trying to help. The kids watching a movie and eating crisps and milling into tins of sweets. Maura had swooped in, lidded the sweets and cooked the dinner, which they'd eaten in stages until late. Melon first, obviously, then potatoes and carrots, turkey almost last of all. It had worked out fine and they'd laughed about it together, all of them, Michelle especially thinking it hilarious that they were having a fifteen-course dinner or whatever it had turned out to be in the end.

'My grandmother was also a bit funny,' Ellie added after a pause.

Declan stroked her hand, which was gripping the edge of the bench.

'I guess all families have different diseases,' he said. 'In mine it's heart attacks. Both my grandads dropped dead when they were in their fifties. I never met them. At least your mum's still around.'

'Well, she is and she isn't.' Ellie turned her hand over and allowed it to be clasped. 'She doesn't remember me. At least I don't think she does. Well, at least I don't think she does all of the time. Sometimes she ...' Ellie paused. Declan kissed her again.

They spent hours painting together, every so often stopping to kiss and surge into each other: the newness of it surprising them, the way desire could pull their bodies together. Maura returned close to teatime when the sun had moved off the wall. Sitting on the bench smiling, she admired their work.

'It's gorgeous,' she told them. 'You're a handy painter, Declan. Aren't we lucky Ellie plucked up the courage to talk to you!'

Ellie blushed hotly, but they were all laughing and she felt happy there in the shade, the colours intensified now the sun's glare had faded.

When Declan went home Maura seemed too exhausted to do anything. Ellie cooked sausages on the grill and made her sit. While the sausages split and sizzled she sliced up a loaf of Bewley's white sandwich bread. Maura was partial to Bewley's and Ellie tried hard to cut the slices evenly the way her aunt liked.

'How is Uncle Pat?' Ellie asked finally, putting plates on the table.

Maura deliberated, holding her face in her hands. 'First my mother, then my sister, and now, perhaps, my brother.' She looked away from Ellie, through the window to the garden and the mural, radiant in the summer evening light. 'It's like seeing flares, these little fragments of genetic material, a pattern emerging ... ah I don't know what I'm saying.' She stopped. Her mind ran through all the instances that in retrospect could have been pointing to what had happened, what was happening to her siblings now: the misplacing of keys, the forgetting of appointments, the times they'd lost their way in familiar places. There was pure despair in having to see those she loved begin to break up, stutter into incoherence, walk towards oblivion.

'When your mum saw our mother was beginning to forget herself,' Maura continued, 'she went to all sorts of talks, read all kind of books. She banished aluminium pans from the house, began doing daily crosswords, ate more broccoli, upped her exercise regime; all the walking. You remember the walking. The sea swimming. But it didn't stop it coming for her, did it? And far earlier than for our mother. All that battling against some misalignment of minuscule particles, hidden away inside. It was all for nothing. At the time Pat said to me it was just plain bad luck. He seemed able to let it go. Of course, he felt sad when he saw her so uncharacteristically angry or strange. When she couldn't remember enough to talk about everyday things. He felt sad for you. But Pat's attitude was always charge on ahead. Think positive. We'll do everything we can for Ellie, he said. We'll manage together. He was cross when we wouldn't go to France with them, wasn't he? Maybe we should have gone.'

Maura was shakier than Ellie had ever seen her before. She reached out to hold her aunt's two hands across the table.

'And now there's a kind of terror in me,' Maura said quietly. 'Today Pat's finally realising that maybe it isn't just bad luck. And I'm seeing that my own chances of getting away unscathed are diminishing, day by day by day.'

*

At the weekend Pat, Anne, and the kids came down to see the mural. The weather was to break the next day, so Maura said they might as well make the most of it and barbeque outside. She made potato salad and coleslaw, rinsed soft lettuce leaves in a basin of salted water. Declan came round early to help Ellie set the table and hull punnets of strawberries bought from a roadside stand: small, perfect berries that stained their fingers and mouths red. After they'd eaten, everyone sat on, enjoying the last of the heat. Ellie and Declan were squashed side by side on a towel. She felt like she was on the edge of the conversation, listening in. She didn't feel that she had to say or do anything so she just stayed sitting there, knowing that eventually the moment would pass away. She noticed Michelle had perched on the arm of the bench beside her dad. She was holding his hand. The others sat on blankets on the yellowing grass. The mural looked glorious. Everyone said so. There was so much colour in it. All through the winter it would lift them each time they looked outside. Even on the greyest, rainiest days, it would bring back memories of the heatwave and the days they'd spent in the sun.

The Portal

Caleb Klaces

One day my father called to tell me he had nowhere to sleep. 'Someone has buried my bed,' he said. It was as though he had played no part in the process. Three months later, he decided to move out. He was going to live with the woman he loved. I knew Jane from my childhood; she and my father had been in a relationship for approximately the first 15 per cent of my adolescence. For some reason he now called her Julia. Jane/Julia lived with her two grown-up sons in a cottage by the sea. The three of them arrived at my father's house in an amber Transporter, fifty-three minutes late. My father had packed a single cloth bag. It contained an apple, a corduroy tie and a sweets tin filled with elastic bands. He explained that he and Julia were going to run a school together. I was concerned about what his hosts were getting themselves into. For a while it might be entertaining to live with a man attempting to teach them and their cheese plants the Year Eight maths curriculum from 1987. But at some point, I predicted, he would need to call on me, as he had so many times before, and I would be 296.6 miles by road (i.e. too far) away.

I looked around the abandoned house. Using a rough visual method, I calculated that in each of the five rooms, he had accumulated an average of 10,000 items. It was not difficult to infer that 50,000 items in total were contained within the walls. If all of these items were placed on one side of an enormous set of scales, it would take some fifty medium-build humans standing on the other side to achieve equilibrium. Instead of other people, however, he had chosen to live with second-hand books, alternative medicines, spent packaging and every imaginable (I exaggerate) type of artefact. There was precisely one item about which I cared. I would have swapped the entire house for it. But there was no one in the world who could tell me where it was.

In the room that had once been my bedroom I sat on the carpet tossing individual copies of *The Journal for Research in Mathematics Education* over my head, enjoying the forlorn sound an old, stiff magazine makes when it hits pebbledash wallpaper. As I did, I revealed, part by enormous cuboid part, my first home computer. I found the power cable and plugged it in. It emitted a syncopated wheezy buzz that was 100 per cent nostalgic (50 per cent pleasure/50 per cent pain). But it also produced a smell that was 100 per cent scorched circuitry. I reprimanded my fifteen-year-old self for failing to release the floppy disk before powering down. I tried it again. This time it lit up. I expected the disk would contain Number Munchers or some vector experiments in Paint. Instead, to my surprise, I found a story.

'The Portal' is about a group of five friends. They live in a small Midlands city (pop. circa 600,000). It is the summer following their first year at sixth form college. None of them has ever swum in the sea. They want more of the world. They construct, accidentally, a machine that functions as a portal into another person's consciousness. The consciousness belongs to an old man named Brian. They know him already. They call him Bitter Brian because he complains to one of them, who is part-time assistant manager of the local supermarket, about everything from the placement of toothpaste in Aisle Eight (illogical) to the decline of singing in the modern world (a conspiracy). The group of five agree they don't like Brian. They imagine the ways they will use their invention to humiliate him. They will make the old man remove his trousers in the lingerie department of the shopping centre. They will make him drink a bottle of cider in Aisle Eight, and then sing.

To their dismay, they soon realise The Portal does not allow them to force Brian to do what they want. They can only enter the machine one at a time. Once inside, nothing of their usual life is present. They have no memories, no intentions and no control. They experience only what Brian experiences. What Brian experiences seems to be a profound and interminable confusion, punctuated by assisted trips to the toilet and dreamless sleep. They take it in turns to 'go senile'. They compete to see who returns from The Portal with the best (i.e. grossest) story.

As term begins again, four out of five of the group turn against the machine. The former supermarket employee switches to working night shifts in a nursing home. She has an average of fifty minutes a day for leisure, which she devotes to the study of C++. The other three decide that The Portal is tedious. They discover weed and then alcohol. In the cinema car park, or the scrub by the railway tracks, or at someone's house when their parents are away, they devote evenings to manufacturing in their bodies a profoundly excited state of confusion, punctuated by assisted trips to the toilet, ending always in dreamless sleep. The following morning, thirsty and sensitive, they laugh nervously about what they remember: who took their trousers off, who woke the neighbours with their singing. They consider themselves one step closer to freedom.

The fifth member of the group keeps The Portal under his bed. Every day after sixth form, he declines the invitation to go along with the others and hurries home to the machine. He does not think of what he is doing as 'going senile'. In fact, he begins to feel ashamed of the phrase. Brian is not confused, the young man decides. Rather, Brian has an extraordinary ability. Brian perceives the wrinkles in space-time smoothed over by ordinary perception. He sees the confusion within the fabric of the universe itself. Brian may be younger in the afternoon than he was in the morning. It may be winter with a bowl of soup and spring with a chocolate biscuit which follows. A father, long dead, steps out from the wardrobe. A war song bubbles up from the kitchen sink. The rough armchair, the blunt razor, the carer's breath: each leaves an impression overwhelmingly tender and lush and uncertain. On returning to his bedroom, the teenager finds his own face covered in salty tears.

One afternoon when the young man is in The Portal, Brian goes out to his front garden to pick blackberries. He washes them in his kitchen sink. His doorbell rings. Brian's chest tightens in anticipation. It is a young woman. Her name is Anita and she is his granddaughter. Brian hands her a bowl of blackberries. She speaks in a slow, deliberate manner. In her company, so does Brian. She laughs. So does he. The blackberries are gone. The chair is empty. Brian looks around the house in a panic. She phones. She will visit again soon. Brian is relieved. He writes himself a note.

Once out of The Portal, the young man is suddenly aware of the vanishingly small number of times in his own life he has glimpsed something real: the morning the cat was eaten by next door's dog; the afternoon he learned of the existence of the decimal point; the night his mother disappeared. All of these moments are eclipsed by what has just happened in The Portal. He has felt a true connection between two people. To care for another person needn't be competitive and humiliating, as his friends would suggest. It can be quiet and generous. It can be as innocent as a bowl of hand-picked blackberries.

But there is a problem. Every time Brian opens the door and sees Anita's face, the young man is aware of an appreciation of her features which is unmistakeably erotic. He is unsettled. In The Portal he only ever feels what Brian feels. Brian appears, therefore, to feel an attraction to his own granddaughter. The young man decides to treat this desire as Brian treats the incomprehensible purple stain on his fingers: he decides to ignore it. But the attraction to the young woman only grows more obvious and persistent. He sees her lips without looking at them. He feels her hands on his face, without her ever touching him. He realises that these cannot be Brian's feelings. They must be his own. It is his desire that runs like a hairline fracture through Brian's familial love. For a moment, he is relieved. Brian's affection remains pure. Then relief turns to anguish. He has spoiled the only true relationship he's ever known.

For the first time he remains in The Portal all night, hoping Brian's sleep will wash through his body and drown the yearning. It doesn't work. In the morning he returns to his bedroom exhausted. It seems pointless and childish to get dressed, to sit for thirty-three long minutes on the bus, to listen for almost an hour to a teacher explain why Lenny is the real hero. He goes back to sleep. In his dream he draws a shape of a thousand and one equal sides. There are so many sides that the shape becomes a circle. Within the circle is a nipple. He shudders awake, sticky and contorted, in cool afternoon spring sunshine. He scrubs himself in the shower, eats a piece of toast, then returns to The Portal. Anita sits close to Brian. Her knees touch his thigh. She lifts out of her bag a small block of pale wood. Brian made her a doll when she was a child. He feels the wood in his (Brian's) hands. His fingers extend out, into the wood itself, and touch a shape inside the grain. The shape lingers as the blade of a red penknife works the wood into a rhyme. He has never known Brian so concentrated, and he feels himself concentrated into a knot, hard and fixed, and understands that the only way to rid himself of his desire is to pursue it.

An entire academic year has gone by since the group of five constructed The Portal. The temperature gradient lifts them suddenly 3°C into summer. The four others, it turns out, are prepared. They have applied themselves to their studies. Their heads are already in other, more interesting cities, where they will soon live. He wakes one afternoon to a deathly silence, with no birdsong, no barking dog, no child playing in the lane, and for a moment, is convinced that he is utterly alone in the world. That evening, he leaves the machine under his bed. He steps outside. He remembers how deeply he dislikes the outside. The tarmac and flickering street lights are like an animal's cage. But Anita is here somewhere, in her body, alive. He goes to a place he remembers her mentioning to Brian. Brian was curious about what people did in a nightclub. She told him she stands up against the enormous speakers and lets them shake her. He finds her there, shaking.

One morning at the end of the summer, he and Anita are sitting on her bedroom floor. He is helping her choose a selection of family photographs to take to visit her grandfather. A lone bird's late love song floats through the open window. He reaches out to touch her shoulder, but recoils. His finger is Brian's finger. His touch is the old man's touch. He goes home and takes a screwdriver to the machine. He leaves The Portal alone for a day, a week, two weeks. He is happy to be close to Anita. Proximity to her is all he needs. Then one evening they watch a film together. It is *Mrs Doubtfire*. Anita is lying down with her legs across his lap. On the screen, Mrs Doubtfire's wig falls off. The deception is becoming clear. Anita gasps and shuffles her body into his. He holds her hand. In his mind, he lays his body down next to hers. His body does nothing.

He storms back to his room and reconstructs The Portal. It is two hours after sunset. Brian is asleep in a chair. The old man stands up, as though woken by the teenager's arrival. He holds a red curtain between finger and thumb and draws it across the window. Brian knows he is closing his curtains yet doubts what he knows. It feels as though he is playing a game. The glass is dark. He can see his own reflection. There is another face inside his reflection. Someone is standing in the brambles and staring in. It is Anita. She holds her arms out, desperate for an embrace. She looks so very sad. Her eyes are holes. Brian accepts the visitor. Perhaps this girl is part of the game. He waves goodbye, closes the curtains and turns towards the stairs. Then he stops. His body is cold with horror. It is the young man's horror, not Brian's. The young man knows Brian can feel it too, and that both of them have been visited by death.

The Portal has changed. The young man is no longer a spectator. He cannot protect Brian from his own feelings. He must make a decision. He chooses to be with Anita. He will tell her, that day, about The Portal. He pledges to destroy the machine. She has something to tell him too. She wants him to meet her grandfather, the one she has told him so much about. He keeps his own secret to himself. He makes his excuses and goes home. Perhaps you do not have to choose after all. Under exceptional conditions, x can also be y. Anita has finally invited him into the most private circle of her life. He doesn't need to renounce The Portal in order for them to be together. In fact, he reasons to himself, if he is happy with Anita (and the balance of probability leans dramatically in his favour), then it is an act of generosity to go into The Portal and transmit his happiness to the old man. Greedily, he returns to his room.

The following day, Anita takes him to meet her grandfather. He wants, more than anything else, to believe this is possible. The outside world is desiccated and colourless. Leaves crunch under their feet. She finds it odd but charming that he is so strongly moved by the walk up Brian's driveway. They reach the front door. He is crying. He tries to explain that she will find a dead body inside the house, but it is not his fault. His mouth will not form the words. He tries to pull her away from the door. She looks at him in bewilderment. She knocks on the door. He is shaking his head and moaning. She has a key. He grabs at her hand, so that she cannot put the key in the lock. She tells him there is nothing to be afraid of. Her grandfather will be happy to meet him. He wipes his face with his sleeve. He looks in her bright, impatient eyes. 'There was immense pain in it,' he tries to explain, 'and almost infinite reluctance, but it was also good.'

This was the end of the story. After the final paragraph, there were three and a half pages of ideas and discarded sentences. Then there was a note I had written to myself.

Gave this to Dad. He printed it off and says he has read it three times. He says the first time he imagined these two people would definitely stay together. The second time he decided that after sharing a loss like that, they could never stay together. Now he isn't sure what he thinks, except that he would like to read more by this talented author.

I turned off the computer. (After ejecting the floppy disk.) I stood in the middle of the room and wondered what I was looking for. My memory of the item returned in increments, like a web page loading on dial-up internet. I looked everywhere. After the best part of two hours (96 per cent?) I gave up. I removed all the rubbish from my father's bed. I slumped, face first, onto the lumpy mattress. Right in front of my eyes, in the space between the frame and the wall, was the object. I picked it up with great care. It was a scale model, in paper and cardboard, of the house in which I was sitting. (The precise scale, it pains me to say, I have forgotten.) I'd constructed the walls and floors and painted the wallpaper. My father had carved the wooden furniture with his red penknife. There were two figures glued in place around the miniature kitchen table. They were drinking tea. As a whole, the model was much less sophisticated than I had remembered. But the two small people touched me deeply.

It was not for my own sake that I had come looking for this childish replica of a forgettable terraced house. It was to benefit my father. My plan was to drive the piece to Jane/Julia's house. Once there, I would place it immediately in front of his face (he was short-sighted and never wore his glasses). Then I would challenge him to see … what? That this was his real home? That this object was proof that Jane/Julia's house was the wrong place for him to be?

I hesitated. The two figures around the table were perfect, I thought. The proportions did not make sense, from a mathematical point of view. But it was undeniable: he and I had made something perfect. To leave my father's house without the two figures would have been, at that moment, the most painful thing I could imagine. I took a deep breath. I replaced the model where he had kept it, among the cobwebs and the yellowed textbooks. I walked through the front door into the sunshine. I imagined him in his new house, looking out of the window at the sea. I imagined he liked it there. I imagined he didn't need me.

Fingerpost

Mary Morrissy

Christine is sitting in her car having a panic attack. At least, that's what she thinks is happening. It's both more and less frightening than she expected. No gasping for breath or throat closing up or heart going like the clappers. No, it's just this. It's 4.30 p.m., a mild February afternoon, the bare trees shrouded in a blurred light, and she hasn't a clue where she is. There's no one about. Even though the street where she has parked, or abandoned herself, is homely with a cottage-style terrace on one side facing a large green, the houses have a stand-offish air, curtains drawn, no cars in the driveways and no evident signs of life.

Enter the Mount Helicon Demesne, the directions had said. When she drove in, it looked like one place, but Mount Helicon was an entire universe. Each development led into another and although the houses changed style, she felt like she was trapped in a Rubik's Cube. Enormous, detached McMansions with mock Tudor beams and double garages gave way to more modest gingerbready two-storeys with dormer windows and curlicued eaves. Then came little courts of maisonettes that were boxy and Swedish-looking – or what Christine imagined as Swedish-looking, since she'd never been there.

Take a right on to Granary Hill, the Google sheet had instructed. She'd driven past a dozen landscaped green spaces, some flat and planted with single, spindly-looking trees, others sloping like the grassy knolls of a golf course. Nothing had appeared that looked like a granary, not to mention a proper hill. It was as if she'd entered a world where the names had no relationship to the landmarks. And it was totally deserted. Not a sinner about. She might as well have been in the Gobi Desert.

She'd been smug starting out. *Head south on Empress Avenue towards Marine Road*. 'I know how to get to the end of my own road,' she'd muttered to herself. When they'd bought the car, Jim had suggested satnav, but she didn't like the idea of a woman in the car, (they're always women, aren't they?) barking instructions at her. 'Don't I have you for that?' she'd said to Jim. Jim's specialty is telling her to turn when it's too late and then getting impatient with her as if she's some kind of dimwit. She savours the experience of driving alone because she neither has to speak nor listen. It's a matter of policy with her that on trips like this, she never brings her mobile. She likes the feeling of being untethered, being in nowhere land, unreachable. That feels transgressive these days.

Veer left onto ramp for Circular Road. Christine had veered as instructed; her whole life is veering just now. Ducking and diving to avoid being side-swiped by the mortifications of ageing. Sniffing her armpits to see has she developed the old-lady smell yet, that perfumed mix of sweet decay she remembers from aunts of long ago: talcum powder, sherry and eau de something like cologne. Who's she codding? She's trying to avoid thinking about death. Delma's kind of death in particular. Delma is her best friend. That sounds meagre and inadequate; her lifelong companion, that's more like it. *Pace* Jim.

Before Delma went into the nursing home, Jim had begun to get tetchy about the amount of time Christine spent with her. Her visits to Delma's increasingly chaotic house took longer and longer, partly because Delma told her everything twice over. There was always a bottle of wine on the go, even if she called in the morning, and when she tried to leave there were scenes.

'Don't go,' Delma would say, clutching her sleeve, 'don't leave me.'

Christine had felt torn, afraid of Delma's drowning grip and dreading Jim's low-lying hostility. All he was worried about was that she was spilling the beans to Delma.

'About our sex lives?' Christine had asked, trying to humour him.

That's what Jim thinks women talk about; even at their age when there's not much going on in that department. But it's intimacy he means. He suspects she might share more of herself with Delma than with him. And that's probably true. Or, at least, it was in the past. Mostly she kept the details of Delma's decline from him. She didn't know why. To protect Delma? But to protect her from what?

Merge onto the South Link, the next command had said. There was a lot of merging in the Google directions. People say that about the elderly; how they merge into the background, become invisible. Not true of Delma, who had become more defined, more definite as she aged. Once she'd given up on colour, her hair underneath turned out to be a majestic and uniform white. She'd acquired a whole new wardrobe. Suddenly she could wear reds and purples because they no longer shouted at her hair. Titian, Delma used to joke, that's the posh name for my shade of carrot. She'd become more flamboyant, buying roomy shift dresses with big pockets and swaddling a pashmina around her neck. A more youthful style than the sober office wardrobe she'd had to wear all her working life. It was a bit mutton dressed as lamb, if you asked Christine, but she said nothing. Now she wonders if this new freedom of expression had been the early signs of Delma's illness taking hold?

Her decline had been so gradual, it was hard to say. It was only when her drinking got out of hand – there'd been some incident with her cleaner – that Delma's niece took charge and moved her into the Mount Helicon Nursing Home.

It had taken Christine months to pluck up the courage to visit. That first time she'd been shocked to see how much weight Delma had lost. Her fingers were too slender to keep on what she used to call her memory ring. She would move it from her left hand to her right to remind her of what she might forget: medical appointments, car repairs, the hair salon. Once Delma would have been delighted with her new slender outline, but Christine doesn't know if such things register with her any longer. Delma had always struggled with her weight and Christine never imagined that in old age *she'd* be the one with the 'fuller figure' – isn't that the euphemism?

When she and Delma were younger they were always going on diets. Scarsdale. Atkins. The soup diet. The grapefruit diet. Christine still weighs herself once a week on the bathroom scales. Her weight flashes up in kilos. She's never got the hang of metric. She memorises the flashing digits, sometimes even writes them down, promising herself she'll convert them into stones and pounds. But even when she's done the conversion, she doesn't act on it. It's a ritual, something she's observed all her adult life. Self-imposed, punitive. At her age, who cares what weight she is?

She hasn't been back to Mount Helicon since that first visit in November. Jim drove her then and she hadn't taken any notice of the route. When she was the passenger, she switched off her interior compass. It was like being a child again, freed of responsibility. Although not freed of worry, given Jim's buccaneering driving. He still drives like he's a young blade, with impatient, showy speed.

That day he'd dropped her at the nursing home and waited outside. When she came out, he was like Patience on a monument, fingers drumming on the steering wheel, and she was irritated with him, given what she had just witnessed. But when she got into the car, she realised he was accompanying the Rolling Stones on the car radio; he was reclaiming his youth and channelling Charlie Watts. He'd asked how Delma was, then started the engine before she could reply.

Continue for 2.4 kilometres ... once on the Link Road, it had been plain sailing for a while. She hugged the inside lane; it felt safer there. Let the speed merchants overtake her. She remembered teaching Delma to drive. Delma had been in her forties before she learned, and, according to one of her many driving tutors, was 'resistant to instruction'. She'd considered it an outrage that she was expected to do various things with her feet, hands, eyes and brain simultaneously. *What am I, a juggler?* Christine remembered accompanying her on the test route many times. (Delma passed on her fourth attempt.) Delma carried on a cranky monologue as she bunny-hopped and ground the gears, excoriating the incompetence of the other drivers. *Look at this, back off buddy, oh no, don't bother to indicate, you know where you're going,* etc. Christine had been shocked. It wasn't road rage, exactly, it was more road peeve. After her last visit to the nursing home, Christine is afraid it's this Delma – Car Delma – who has the upper hand.

She had come with a large bouquet of flowers, wrapped in a cellophane trumpet. A carer, a bosomy young woman in blossomy scrubs, who introduced herself as Sara, met her in the foyer and offered to take her to Delma's room. They'd travelled down the blush-coloured corridor, passing an open area where a group of residents was gathered, some in wheelchairs, others enveloped by soft chairs. They looked like they were waiting for something to happen.

'We're expecting a fortune teller,' Sara said in explanation.

Really, Christine had thought, couldn't they work out for themselves what the future held?

'Delma, you've got a visitor!' Sara announced as she held the door open to let Christine pass. She was just in time to see Delma make a sour face like a bold child and then immediately readjust it by putting on a wide smile.

It was a big, airy room with a large picture window, a view of a distant mountain, snow-veined at the peak. Christine immediately thought of a Swiss sanatorium. Newly thin Delma was propped up on a number of pillows, looking straight at her. She was engulfed by a teal-coloured candlewick dressing gown. Christine remembered it from holidays: Delma wrapped in it, slopping out on to the balcony to light up and inhale the balmy Mediterranean night along with the nicotine. Those holidays had been like small draughts of freedom, away from Jim and the kids. Delma abroad was always so extravagant, buying outsized ceramic bowls that had to be hawked back on the plane, and ordering exotic cocktails with umbrellas, without knowing the ingredients. Despite her colouring, she loved the sun, drank it up, while Christine stuck to the shade.

'Jesus!' Delma had said, eyeing the flowers, 'who's dead?'

Christine was taken aback. Delma never used to swear. In the car, she might have called other drivers cretins in her exhalations of scorn but she'd never taken the Lord's name in vain. She'd been quite strait-laced like that.

'It's me, Delma,' she'd said.

'You're dead?' Delma said looking her up and down coolly.

'No, I mean ...'

'I know who the hell you are, Chris, I'm not completely gaga.'

She'd placed the flowers on the table tray and sat down beside the bed. For the next twenty minutes they'd had a routine conversation, small talk about Jim and the boys.

Delma had never married. In the early eighties, there'd been a short engagement to Eddie Cloney, a dapper, reckless guy who wore three-piece suits and had a weakness for the gee-gees. Not exactly husband material, Delma said. But then, Christine had always felt Delma wasn't exactly wife material. She'd never got the whole story about Eddie, and she'd never asked, because it felt like prying and Delma had been very cut up about it. See, Jim, female friendship isn't all about blabbing. There are things we don't talk about.

'And how's my god-daughter?' Delma asked.

Christine's daughter Trudy was in the States. An image of her daughter had floated into Christine's head, an old image of her when she was a teenager, her long dark hair swirled up on top of her head, like she is in the framed photo on the piano. Like she was before the two hard-won babies – fertility problems, there's an irony – the ranch house in Cupertino, the tech-wizard American husband with the good teeth. When she was a teenager, Trudy had affected not to care much for Delma. But when Christine and Trudy had gone through their bad patch, it was to Delma that Trudy had turned.

'I told her,' Delma had said vehemently at the time, 'that you were my friend first and I wouldn't countenance seeing you put down.'

Christine remembered flushing with pride at this statement. But when she'd pressed Delma about what Trudy had said about her, Delma had been very firm. She wouldn't reveal what she'd been told in confidence.

'Trudy's fine,' Christine said, wanting to add, 'as far as I know.'

Their weekly Skype calls, which should have helped with the distance, made Christine feel more estranged. Sometimes, she longed for the plain old landline call. Just voice, no pictures, no performance required. When Trudy and Mike came home, it was the same. It wasn't that she didn't love it when they were here, but she was always relieved that American holidays were so short. They usually only stayed a week or two. Christine couldn't bear the intimacy of it all the time – the chaos of two kiddies, close in age, trapped in a new environment, her daughter's laissez-faire style of mothering, Mike's effervescent optimism. He was a hands-on father and sometimes Christine felt even that was a rebuke to her. Jim had never so much as changed a nappy when hers were babies.

The antics of the American visits mostly passed Jim by. He would whisk Trudy off at some point to get her on her own, leaving Christine with Mike and the kids. 'Let your mother play the granny,' he'd say, or words to that effect, 'she loves it.' But Christine didn't. She'd never bonded with those children: she was wary of them, and they made strange with her. She couldn't get over her resentment that they spoke with American accents. They didn't sound like her, or Trudy. It was as if they didn't belong, as if they were cuckoos in the nest. But she couldn't say that, now could she?

A familiar landmark appeared – the Fingerpost Roundabout. In the central island, there was an old-style signpost painted white with the destinations printed in hand-done black lettering and a medieval-sleeved hand with its fingers elegantly pointing at the arrow-shaped tips. But when she looked at the Google directions there was no mention of the Fingerpost. The roundabout had four exits and Google said to veer left. But which left? At least two of these were left. Maybe she was approaching the roundabout from the wrong side? She thought of the Irish joke about directions – *I wouldn't start from here, love.* She drove around the Fingerpost three times, trying each of the exits, but was forced to turn back each time since the Google directions didn't match what she was seeing. Well, she thought, that was the beauty of roundabouts; you could keep going around until you got it right. But she was cross with herself. She knew this place, it was only twenty minutes from home as the crow flies, but after she'd driven around it three times she felt like she'd submitted to some ancient superstitious ritual and entered another dimension.

'I've never liked Trudy,' Delma said.

'What?'

'No,' Delma had corrected herself, 'I *used* to like her, but I don't like how she turned out. I mean your boys …'

Christine had smiled to herself thinking of Phelim and Tim. Loyal to their mother, they'd never given her a moment's worry.

'Well, let's face it, they were always plodders,' Della ploughed on. 'But Trudy, Trudy had spirit and you stifled it.'

Delma watched her with those same candid blue eyes she'd known since they were teenagers. Since they were Chris and Del, mending their denims and having their hearts broken. They'd had their spats. Christine recalled a month's silence over a borrowed dress that got ripped at a charity disco, and another feud about a boy one of them fancied and the other one went out with. It was so long ago now that Christine couldn't even remember which way round it was. But she'd never doubted the fact of their friendship. Now she wasn't so sure.

With Delma, the social brakes seemed to be off.

Or was it the gloves?

'I mean the way you behaved about the baby business. She told me that you wouldn't hear of her keeping it …'

What was Delma doing, dragging up ancient history like this?

'It was for her own good, it would have held her back, ruined her life.'

'Nonsense, Christine, you couldn't bear it. Sending her off like that.'

Christine didn't like the way Delma was appropriating her name, like a cold-caller. And since when had she become Christine? And she hadn't sent Trudy off anywhere; that made it sound like she'd dispatched her to a Magdalene laundry.

'I told her not to do it,' Delma said. 'If you really want to know.'

Christine didn't.

'I told her she should stand up to you.'

'I thought you were on my side,' Christine said.

'Whatever made you think that?'

So much for 'you're my friend first'. Christine found herself spluttering. 'Because, because ...'

'You could have helped with the baby, Chris, and that way Trudy could have had it all. I mean it was the nineties, not the dark ages.'

No one, Christine thought, could have it all.

'She was a child herself,' Christine said.

'All the more reason for you to be the adult,' Delma snapped.

'So, if you felt this strongly, why didn't you ever say anything about it before?'

'It wasn't my place,' Delma said.

'But it is now?'

Was this the illness talking? Or was this what Delma had felt all along? In the past she'd often been sharpish, with a hard, glittery edge. Now she was a sword unsheathed.

Delma shrugged, eyeing her dubiously.

'It was the best thing, Del. It gave her a second chance,' she said, hearing the appeasing tone in her own voice, even though she was livid.

Delma didn't know what she was talking about. Delma hadn't been there when Christine arranged for Trudy to stay with a nice Catholic family in Dublin, where she earned her keep by looking after the woman's children. It was a nice family home. Delma wasn't the one who got the doctor to certify Trudy's absence from school (colitis, a condition to which no blame could attach), so that she'd have a clean record when she went back to do her repeats and no one would be any the wiser. Trudy could never have organised all that on her own. And all without her precious father realising. She'd told him Trudy had got a Transition Year placement in Dublin. He'd swallowed that fiction, never questioned it once, because in his eyes, his precious Trudy could do no wrong.

'Look at her now!' Christine said hotly.

'Yeah,' Delma said, 'exactly. She ran away as soon as she could. You taught her to do that. She's a mirror image, settling for less, not to mention the idiot husband ...'

'Excuse me ...'

She wanted to slap Delma, right across the face, a sharp smack.

'And always so tightly wound up. When they come home, my God, Trudy's on a wire spring all the time. So busy pretending. Just like you. Look at you now,' Delma said pointing to Christine's hands, which were clenched in fists of rage on her lap. 'You don't know how to let go.'

I *have* let go, she'd wanted to shout. I've been letting go all my life. Didn't I let Trudy to go off to the States on her own after the other business, even though all I wanted was to cling on to her and protect her, though she didn't need it, and the thing she needed protecting from had already happened. And if I'm not letting go, I'm thinking of how I'll do it when the time comes, with Jim, and myself. And you, Delma.

'You've been a terrible mother to her, Chris, and what's more ...'

She had to put a stop to Delma's gallop. She'd inhaled deeply.

'And what exactly would you know about mothering, Delma?'

Christine was getting hot under the collar, literally. Long after menopause, she still suffered phantom hot flushes as if the body was secretly addicted to fire. Fourth time around the Fingerpost, she careened on to the only route left to her, desperately looking for the next turn, which should be on the left, after eighty-six metres. Metric measure again. How far was that? She had no idea. But not far, she guessed. But there was no turn at all on the left and a mile had gone up on the clock. She slowed down. The car behind her flashed. She was really sweating now, armpits sticky. She started to rage against the useless directions, shouting to herself inside the car, spittle flying. She was still fulminating when she came upon another roundabout. The driver behind pulled up level with her as they halted to let traffic go by. He was a young man with a crew cut and she was aware of him watching her sidelong. Crazy old bird, that's what he was thinking as he roared off, leaving her behind.

She hugged the inside lane and chugged all the way around to go back to the Fingerpost. She picked the first route she had tried even though she was pretty sure it couldn't be right. She was pretty sure everything about this visit was doomed now. And yet she drove on blindly.

In the end, she found the Mount Helicon estate by chance. She'd passed it several times and thought, no it can't be in there, that's just a housing estate. But the name gave her hope. She plunged into the estate and that was when she really lost her bearings.

There had been a long silence before Delma reacted.

'Duck,' she cried, 'it's Magda!'

'Who?' Christine said half rising from her chair and turning towards the door where she expected one of the carers to appear. Meanwhile Delma was sitting up rigid in the bed, flapping her hands about, bowing low then rearing up as if under attack. Then she remembered. Magda was Delma's cleaner who came once a week when she couldn't keep up with the housework. It was Magda who'd alerted Delma's niece that she really wasn't managing. At the time, Christine felt foolish that she hadn't realised how far gone her friend was.

'The crow,' Delma said, raising her voice and putting her hands to her ears.

'What crow?' Christine asked, though she was scouring the room following Delma's wavering eyes as the bird dive-bombed about the room. Once in the early days of their marriage, a collared dove had got caught in the kitchen and Christine had nearly lost her mind. It was a summer's afternoon, and it flew in the back door, which was thrown open. In its panic it had swooped and squawked. She'd flapped a tea towel at it. Jim had said, no, stop, you'll only make it worse, but Christine was afraid it might attack her, go for her eyes. That was the trouble with trapped birds: they were terrified and terror-inducing. Christine had wanted to run out of the house, let the bird have the place, but Jim said, don't do anything, just sit down and ignore it. How could she ignore it, this feral creature veering about the kitchen, crashing into the dresser, then the window, and leaving spatters of bird shit all over the floor? It couldn't seem to see the open back door through which it had flown. Christine remembered the term birdbrain.

'Open the window,' Delma cried.

Even as she stood and reached for the latch, Christine found herself rationalising the situation – if the window was closed how did the bird get in? – but Delma's terror was such that she didn't question her. She'd opened the window but when she turned to look at Delma, she could tell from the look on Delma's face that the bird had not left the room. It was still buzzing, it was obviously at Delma's hair. She'd pulled the pillow down over her head and was cowering now, wild-eyed.

'Don't just fucking stand there,' Delma shouted, 'get help!'

Christine hesitated; how would she explain at the nurses' station that she needed assistance to get rid of an imaginary bird?

'You know what it means if you let the effing thing die in here?'

'What?' Christine asked, playing for time.

'Can't you guess?' Delma had said. 'God, I'd forgotten how slow you are on the uptake.'

Delma had never spoken to her like this before and frankly, Christine was afraid of her now. She tiptoed towards the door, as if the fiction of the bird had taken hold of her. She didn't want any of her movements to add to the panic. Just as she reached the door, it opened, and Sara, the carer who'd shown Christine in, appeared with an orange drink in her hand. Christine was frozen in mid-tiptoe and Delma was buried under the bedclothes, only her hair showing.

'Is it Magda again?' Sara asked matter of factly.

She set down the drink on the radiator cover and opened both the top and the side windows, letting in an icy chill. She lifted a blanket from the end of Delma's bed and shook it out, holding it like a curtain in front of her as she moved towards the window. Delma was peering out from under the pillow. Sara narrated her journey as she herded the bird towards escape. 'I'm leading her to the window, Delma, we're nearly there ...'

Delma had unwound herself from behind the pillow.

'Are you sure?'

'Yes, Delma, I'm the expert, remember?'

She went to retrieve the drink. 'Now, Delma, sundowner time!'

Delma's face lit up, the bird crisis forgotten.

'It's my secret tipple!' Delma said, and drank greedily from the beaker. 'Here,' she offered, 'you try it.'

'No,' Christine said, 'no, I'm fine. That's for you.'

'For fuck's sake, Christine, what are you saving yourself for?'

'Now Delma,' Sara said, 'maybe it's too early for your friend.'

Too late, more likely.

'It has vodka,' Delma said.

'Really?' Christine had looked to Sara.

'Oh yes,' Sara said with a minute shake of her head to Christine, 'every patient gets a vodka and orange before dinner.'

When she'd left, Delma put the glass down. 'Awful muck! They only wave the vodka bottle at it. And no nibbles.'

'I'd complain to management,' Christine said, as if they were talking about bad service in a restaurant.

'Oh, don't worry, Chris, I intend to. And if I don't get satisfaction, I'll take my custom elsewhere!'

Christine even managed to smile: this was more like the Delma she knew.

'Remember that awful hotel in Portugal?' Delma said, 'remember, I found a hair on the toilet seat and got us an upgrade?'

They were returned to the calm waters of nostalgic reminiscence.

There's a sharp rap on the car window like the beak of a bird. Christine jumps. She has the heater on and the car has steamed up. She can only see the blurry flesh outlines of the face peering in at her. She wipes a face-shaped patch in the condensation and sees a man of her own age, in a black beanie, peering in. She releases the window switch. As the glass winds down, she notices the man has a dog at his feet. A small little thing, black, smooching up against his ankle like an amorous cat.

'Is everything alright in there?' he asks. What does he think she's doing, a seventy-year-old woman sitting in her car alone at dusk? He has shaggy eyebrows and rimless glasses and a smirky smile that might once, long ago, have been gamey.

Before she has a chance to deny she needs help, her default position, she says quickly 'I'm lost.'

She grabs the Google directions, and jabs at Granary Hill, where she's supposed to turn right.

He takes the page from her and pushes up his glasses to examine it closely.

'Never heard of it,' he says. 'Where are you trying to get to?'
'The nursing home.'

'Ah well now, I know where that is,' he says and thrusts the useless paper back at her. 'You're almost there. Go back to the junction just here, left on to the main drag there and first left. You can't miss it.'

With the afternoon I'm having, Christine thinks, I could easily miss it.

The dog is whining at the man's trouser leg now. He looks at her bashfully as if the mutt has thwarted a romantic tryst.

'Thank you,' she says, and she feels a surge of gratitude to be saved from her ridiculous panic.

The little dog hares off and Mr Beanie goes after him. Thankfully, he's so distracted that he doesn't look back to see if Christine has followed his directions. He takes a rutted track into a copse of trees that divides this street from the next and is gone.

Still, Christine sits there.

She's probably too late now. They'll be having their tea at Mount Helicon. Why is it that meals are served at nursery hours in these places? If it's feeding time, they won't welcome visitors. Better this way, really, Christine thinks. She can make up a story for Jim; he'll never suspect a thing. That part doesn't bother her but letting Delma down feels like betrayal. Then she remembers the last visit. She turns the ignition in the car. She'll make her way back to the Fingerpost roundabout. Once there, she'll be in familiar territory, and she can pretend that none of this has happened. Next time she'll know exactly how to reach Delma without any confusion.

If there is a next time.

Immurement

Sinéad Gleeson

Although it isn't true, I have always thought of my mother as a widow. I can picture a morning, clouds clotted with rain, when a sleek black hearse pulls up outside the house. Someone, an aunt or a neighbour, peels back the net curtain, placing a reassuring hand on her arm and says, 'It's time.' Four men in black suits, affable, wordless, used to the polite routines around death. They shepherd mourners into another room while they perform the final grim ritual of screwing on the coffin lid. I'm wearing the one good blouse I own, neat black trousers instead of a skirt, because it will be cold when it is time for us to gather a fistful of wet soil and throw it into the grave.

My mother is not a widow, even though my father has been long gone. The North for a bit, then the Isle of Man. We think he owns a pub in Manchester now. It was these imagined funereal thoughts that caused me to burn that same good blouse this morning. The iron left a rust-coloured chevron where the heart should be. But it wasn't really my mother's fake widowhood or my father's whereabouts that caused the problem. I was thinking of the man I'd spent many afternoons with last year while his wife was at work. His favourite thing was to rip open that blouse. Afterwards, I would crawl around on the floor searching for the buttons to sew back on. The man did not work. He had family money. But those hours ... filled to the brim with the combined square footage of our flesh. I always left with an angry streak of carpet burn on my back.

Memories of those burns led to the iron burn, and the ultimate ruination of my blouse. The irony is that I never iron anything, not even the blouse-as-prop ahead of those lustful afternoons. But today I will meet with my mother's doctors and a certain amount of effort is required.

My father was a serial cheater. Other people's wives, women he worked with, one neighbour. You couldn't even leave him with a babysitter. I often wonder if I'd inherited his insatiableness. Or maybe just his cruelty. We both felt indifferent about my mother. In some ways it was a blessing that she couldn't remember a lot of it now. How awful he'd been. We didn't miss him.

My mother complains about the noise on the ward. She forgets why she's here sometimes, and each spoon rattling on a saucer, each beeping machine, alerts her to the fact that this is not home. I bought noise-cancelling headphones and downloaded an app on her phone that plays soothing sounds: a Japanese garden, rain falling on a tent, waves at the coast.

The sea always makes me sad, she declared one afternoon.

At this, uncharacteristically, she welled up. I'd only seen her cry a couple of times. Once when her mother died, and again during some unspecific crisis involving my father. This can't be true though. Back then, there was a lot of crying and yet this one homogenised scene is all that I can recall. Before – before the illness – nothing moved her. Not babies, or weddings, sad endings to films, orchestral music. This new late-stage sentimentality took some getting used to.

I bring things from home to brighten up the disinfectant gloom of the ward. She moves further and further away from language and I'm aware that no amount of favourite cups or books will halt this. I want her to feel … not recognition, that is unfair. Recognition is too much of an ask lately. Comfort, maybe. Relief. To see her face break into that tilted, toothed thing she did with her mouth that used to make me feel everything would be ok, even when it wouldn't.

It was a simple procession of offerings: rich, oily hand creams, all on the citrus spectrum: lemon, bergamot, bitter orange; a photo of Dubhín, her black mutt of uncertain heritage who barks a lot, emitting plumes of halitosis, and is disdainful of every living creature except my mother. The objects are a source of conversation for as long as she can hold the thin thread of it. Sometimes, there was a row, usually when she'd stoked around in the furnace of her memory and could find no match for it from her life. Another day, I brought bourbon biscuits – her favourite – and asked Piotr, who brings the tea around, to slip one onto her saucer as a surprise. He made a great ceremony of presenting the tray – there was even a flourish – but the biscuit was regarded with suspicion. Piotr moved to the door and gave a polite bow. A tattoo peered from under his uniform sleeve. He emitted, as always, a clean smell of soap. Mother kept staring at the biscuit. Anxious, I took the packet from my bag, holding up the striped wrapper, hoping it might click.

Why did you bring these?

Her face curdled, collapsing in on itself.

They're your favourites. Bourbon Creams. Remember?

I hate them. I don't know why you brought them. Are they meant for someone else?

The lone biscuit sat on the saucer. I waited.

Unless, of course, you're trying to poison me. Someone else in here is.

She lunged at the packet and threw them – I'm certain – with the specific aim of hitting me. But her muscles were long weakened, her arms constrained by a different kind of atrophy to the one taking place in her mind.

I picked up the remnants, glad Piotr wasn't there to see this. Outside it was getting dark, and despite the hellish seal of the windows, the evening buses could be heard rumbling below, packed with tired commuters. She gazed over my head at the TV, as though nothing had happened, the evening news rattling through bad headlines. A minister in trouble. A teenage boy charged with a knife attack. Farmers protesting climate change curbs.

The women in the other beds had no visitors, but it was still early. Maureen, in the bed nearest the toilet, is often found wandering the corridors saying she needs a lift to meet a fella in town. Next to her is Angelique, who complains about her husband never visiting – *He's a bollix, a waster, after all I've done for him* – A nurse explained to me that her husband has been dead for years.

The days are long, so I read while my mother sleeps, her small limbs twitching. I've been reading books about immurement, the idea of sealing a person into a place with no exits, either as punishment or sacrificial offering. Stories of children bricked into the walls of churches; skeletons found in hidden rooms in buildings. Cause of death was either lack of air or starvation. In Rome, Vestal Virgins tended a sacred fire that was not allowed to go out. As a result of their status, the women were exempt from marriage and procreation. They took a thirty-year vow of chastity and were punished with immurement if they broke it. I read on, about robbers in ancient Persia bricked into walls for their crimes, fascinated by Elizabeth Báthory de Ecsed, a sixteenth-century Hungarian countess who killed hundreds of young girls and was nicknamed the Blood Countess. As punishment, she was immured in a castle for the last years of her life.

Most of the book is scandalous, voyeuristic even, but one chapter moves me immensely. In some cultures, a living person was entombed with a dead loved one so they would not be alone. It seemed to me so unbearable, yet oddly touching.

Piotr interrupts these thoughts with tea, offering us both a cup, eyeing the cover.

Some light reading?

I immediately attempt to alleviate the idea that I'm not a weirdo who likes reading about people being bricked up.

It's for a project I'm working on. (This is a lie.)

Oh, yes?

Learning how to seal terrible people into walls.

He laughs.

Bricks are expensive, no?

So I hear …

Where I come from there is a story like this. I will ask my mother.

If it doesn't sound too creepy, I look forward to it.

He is tall and very thin, but muscular. I imagine him running a lot or doing triathlons. There is something innately hardy about him; I imagine that hopping off a bike and jumping into a deep, green lake would be no bother to him.

***

The illness brought a new frankness to Mother. Harsh statements. Outlandish judgements on others. Questions she'd never dare ask in the past. As I peeled an orange for her, she looked at me for a long time.

How many people have you slept with?

It was interesting that she didn't say men. I definitely considered myself straight but there'd been a couple of women in the past. The actual number? I couldn't honestly say. A figure appeared in my mind, the hum of it. Three hundred? No – could it be four hundred? Maybe I should have been appalled by the discrepancy of a hundred. It wasn't like losing change down the side of the couch. By some people's standards, it was an extremely significant number. But I wanted it to be higher. I was working on it.

Not that you should be asking, but average. Fewer than ten.

She chews the pulpy flesh, making elaborate sucking sounds.

Your Auntie Gráinne cheated on Uncle Mick. Years ago. Said it was great, but it fizzled out. Are there more oranges?

I peel another in silence, citrus stinging a paper cut I didn't know I had.

The stasis of the ward – outside of temperature checks and meals and Piotr, with his kind face, bringing the tea – begins to impose its routines on me. I develop a habit of looking out the window at exactly the same time every day. If I am here in the afternoon, it has to be 3.33 p.m. There is no particular reason. I just like the curved uniformity of the numbers. Three backing singers in a 1960s band. On evening visits, I aim for 7.25 p.m., just before her favourite programme starts.

Tonight's high moon is a taunt. Arrogant, lounging on a blanket of indigo.

I'll be here long after you, but you … what's your contribution to the world? I radiate, I shine, I am the muse of poets. You fuck, and are fucked. You are tawdry and ephemeral.

This is what I imagine the moon says to me most nights.

***

When I was younger, she had such a big circle of friends. Women who looked out for each other, especially ones that didn't have husbands on the scene. The gang she worked with. Agnes from the shop. The ladies she knew from the park and walking Dubhín, and Nora, who she always referred to as a 'lady doctor'. We were talking about Nora the first time I noticed something was wrong. We were having lunch in a small café near the canal, and she was talking about Nora's job, even though I already knew what she did.

She's a doctor of … what's it called, Christ, you know … all that stuff. She drew circles, pointing vigorously downwards.

A gynaecologist?

Yes, I know that. I told you already.

For a brief moment, terror clouded her face. Incomprehension at why the word refused to appear. As a distraction, I joked about how Auntie Pat used to call Nora 'the gee doctor', but she didn't laugh.

I've inherited the dog now, who is like her: elderly and sleeps a lot. I've never had a pet and don't really want one, but I don't have the heart to give her to a shelter. Every morning I take a photo of Dubhín and send it to my mother. Most days I can see she hasn't read the message.

When I arrive today there is an argument in progress. Betty, one of the cleaners, is in the corridor with a face like thunder. The ward sister is soothing my mother, who is addled and crying.

She'd rob the sun to warm her bones! I'm telling ye! BITCH! That one'd take the eye out of your head! Give them back, you BITCH!

Betty is accused of stealing her headphones. They are nowhere to be seen. My mother has shouted the ward down, waking Mrs Murray, who I have never seen awake in all my visits. Hot air is circulated 24/7 into a mattress to keep her from getting bedsores, varicose veins, or some other ailment. It rises and falls like a chest. More alive than its cadaverous occupant.

When they take my mother for a shower, I find the headphones tangled in the bedsheets. Helping her back into bed afterwards, her legs are a shock. Blue-white, completely hairless, the skin has a pearly sheen. All muscle mass gone.

Last year, I slept with a footballer a few times. The only things in his fridge were beer and packets of chicken fillets, sweating under the clingfilm.

***

Tonight, I am wearing an old coat of hers. A gorgeous astrakhan with silky fake fur that I used to borrow as a teenager. We fought about it a lot, from me never asking permission to the fact that it made me 'look older'. I thought it might give us something to talk about, but when I walked in wearing it, she didn't say a word.

The ward is in an old part of the hospital. It's not exactly decrepit, but it's far from TV-hospital shiny. It has a kind of faded grandeur in the architraves, the wide wooden staircase, the high windows over the door frames. If it wasn't for the smell of hot-plated food and sanitiser, it might be mistaken for stately. There is one TV for six patients, above an old radiator, a Victorian-looking thing that hisses regularly. *Sss-sss-sssh*. A reminder of 'Hespis', a word my father used to say, hissing it at her. It always sounded so vicious. There were other words too, that required him to flex his jaws or caused a certain corrugating of his cheeks.

It wasn't until years later on a TV quiz show that I learned it was actually 'Hesperus', and my father was equating my mother to a wreck. It was from a poem by Henry Wadsworth Longfellow. A name, she used to say in a fancy English accent to make me laugh. A posh name. Not like Byrne, or Daly, or Doyle. Double-barrelled names from certain postcodes and schools.

I eye the rain outside, rueing the coat and my decision to cycle, but I couldn't afford a cab. Not after the big night out at the weekend when I'd dusted the coat off for its vintage glamour. The stupid, overpriced cocktails, paltry and insufficiently strong. Taxis to two parties, and another one to find a late-night garage for cigarettes at 2 a.m. That moment on the South Circular Road when I'd leaned against the cool glass of the passenger window, orange street lights splashing across my face. I should have called it a night then. Ghosted. Irish-goodbye-d. Gotten home at a less alarming hour, woke with more money and no one else in my bed. Instead, the next morning had felt like the apocalypse, prising apart dried-on mascara. Skin like tarmac. The curtains had snagged on a chair and a shaft of sun suddenly illuminated a stranger's chest, rippling with shallow breaths. It was almost religious. Pieta-like – without Mary – in sombre olive shades. I don't want to think about that bed, while sitting next to Mother in hers. But I remember us laughing, bumps of ketamine, a glass of red wine knocked over, spilling like a shotgun wound across the floor. There was the feel of his weight, my arm anchored to his back. I was miles away when I felt something on my arm. My mother, wordlessly rubbing the astrakhan sleeve, a soft smile on her lips.

***

The vending machine in the corridor is spectral. Drinks and wrappers in garish shades trapped behind glass. Mother likes those crinkled crisps so I feed the machine coins and watch the packet jump off the shelf like a diver. Piotr comes through the double doors, flushed but smiling. I press cancel and stand aside, gesturing that he go first.

Thank you.

No bother, I'm in no rush.

How are you?

I'm good. You?

Very well, thank you. I asked my mother about the story.

Which story is that?

About the people in the walls back home.

What did she say?

There was a woman the local bishop thought was a witch who had bewitched the local children. There were stories about her trying to get the kids to kill their parents by putting things in their food.

Wow. Sinister.

The real story is that the bishop had gotten this woman pregnant and wanted to keep it quiet.

Ah, a tale as old as time.

It's very wrong. So cruel.

He retrieved a drink, and put more coins in the slot. A pink chocolate bar fell into the drawer below, which he handed to me.

I'm ok, I don—

Your mother. She likes these pink ones. Sorry about the biscuit thing the other day.

And then he was gone, runners squeaking on the vinyl tiles.

When I get back to the ward, she is watching a drama on TV. Maureen is snoring loudly. A woman on screen is begging a politician to help her addict son. My mother seems moved by this, her eyes glistening. I put the pink bar in the drawer of her locker, and she touches my arm.

Women are always the ones up to their neck in it, aren't they? Struggling, trying to get by. And if you stand up for yourself, you're a mouth, or a total weapon. By God, we needed our little groups through. The marches. Spitting feathers over cups of tea. I used to wonder – maybe you'd know? – is there some sort of Freemasons that's just for women? I'd join that, I would. Sign me up. Wait – maybe that's nuns. Or witches – are they still a thing? Like a coven kind of thing. Aye …

Aye. It's a long time since she'd said that. After my father, she'd desperately tried to reinvent herself, working hard to sieve certain vowels out of her voice.

I could hear his voice again. The hard consonants. The local vernacular of put-downs.

TARGER.

SLEEVEEN.

GEEBAG.

On those nights where I am sling-shotted back to the past, the air evaporates from my lungs. I have to get outside. In the foyer there's a full-size religious crib. It seems out of date these days. Joseph has the look of Parnell about him. The dark brown beard carved in relief plastic. Mary's pregnant belly is remarkably flat, even though she's surely only evacuated Himself onto the stable straw. The porcelain arc of her cheekbone is pious, but utterly 1940s Hollywood too. The artist has pinked and glossed her lips, adding a definite hint of the erotic. Mary looks decidedly up for it. Paper lantern lights are strung up over the doors and I recognise them from a chain store. They trot them out in different shades for various occasions: green for St Patrick's Day, black and orange for Halloween, and now a deep scarlet for Christmas. The shade of red is almost unseemly in a hospital.

Outside, I feel the weight of what's happening acutely. It isn't how it's meant to go. How are these things meant to actually go? There is no plan, no blueprint. Sometimes there is just bad luck, hovering over a bed on the third floor. Two snails are fucking on the wall near the bike rack. I watched a nature programme one night after an evening in the pub. It explained that snails were hermaphrodites. Each coupling involves two penises, two vaginas and some sort of love dart. Before all this anatomical swapping, they woo each other and then stick together for hours. It's passive, but oddly touching. Watching their united shells suddenly calls up a loneliness that verges on hysterical.

The snails are not the reason I agreed to meet ketamine man again. It's almost Christmas and a festive drink seems like an acceptable means of participation. People love this time of year: family, heaving plates of succulent meat, day drinking.

Only the external things appeal to me. The way the town glams up: lights swinging on wires, sparkly objects in windows. The sheer excess of festivity, filling up every molecule of air; it is hard not to get sucked in. This will be the first year without our tiny family dinner. No paper hats from crackers or *It's a Wonderful Life.* No brandy and Baileys all day.

On the way to meet him, I try to feel solidarity with the other revellers. The buses heave with young, glossy women, teetering on spiked heels with mermaid-waved hair. Not a single coat covering the cheap glitter of their dresses. *Not a coat.* My mother seeps into my larynx, ventriloquising. When I'm not by her bed, I imagine her soul casts off her body and rises up to follow me around the city, annoyed that I'm not with her. Or maybe this is not the case at all. This act of shadowing is merely a chance to whisper something she always meant to say, but never got around to it.

It's short, my love. Soak it up, soak it up.

The next day I ask how she is feeling and after a long silence that's almost a full stop, she offers one word.

Polluted.

The illness is a burst pipe in the brain, effluvia covering up all the usual routines, recognition, all the words she loved. Tincture. Banjaxed. Effluvia was a good word too. Luxurious, lyrical. At odds with its meaning.

This morning, I also feel polluted. A toxic hangover from the previous night's date, which was only survivable with another bottle of wine. It brought a kind of thin-skinned shell shock; waves of horror floating up through the skin. All the things I'd wanted to do in the past, the places I thought I would go yet found myself sidelined by distractions and time-wasting, stupid behaviour. I'd never had a plan. Too many ordinary days or maybe too much wildness. Vehemence, where were you when I needed you?

At the vending machine, I chug a bottle of Lucozade and make for the door. The lover snails are nowhere to be found. A woman wearing a dressing gown is smoking a cigarette and screaming into a phone. It begins to rain again, and I think of Achill and the lone childhood holiday we took. A funfair near the strand, wind whipping up Keam beach. Everyone talking about a basking shark in the bay though we never saw it. My mother looked content then, rather than happy. Happiness was not something we took for granted and aspiring to it was just asking for trouble. We built a fort in the sand and lay on a tartan blanket, eating crisp sandwiches until all the blue drained out of the sky.

When I go back up to the third floor she is sleeping fitfully, her mouth drooping to one side. A pale blue envelope written in an elegant hand is propped against the cold teacup. The fada is missing, of course, but then he isn't from here. I don't know how to write characters in his language. What is lost when those swirls and lines are omitted? Something glottal, certainly. Maybe something more immense.

Basildon Bond. Old school. I used to write reams of it to a German pen pal. Her letters were long monologues about the food she ate or answering questions about the Rhine. She'd use fancy paper covered in pineapples or girls on roller-skates in pastel greens and pinks.

The letter is a surprising act of formality, of chivalry, even. I wonder if he bought the paper just to write to me and imagine him idling in the stationery section of the newsagent's, wondering if blue said something more than white. Piotr has never mentioned where exactly he's from in his home country. Somewhere really remote maybe, with sporadic broadband. Or perhaps his mother is authoritarian, tough, and refuses to read emails, insisting on handwritten letters, just to see her son's long, sloping hand on a blue rectangle. I wonder if he misses her. How often they speak. If her health is good.

The letter suggests dinner on Saturday. I do not say a word of this to my mother who, in the past, would have had plenty to say about it. A good deal of the time she sleeps now. Eye sockets silken, almost silver, two coins on her face. The change in her breathing is more apparent, a deep clawing for breath.

When she is awake, she talks about me as if I am not there. What I mean is, she speaks to me as if I am another person, not her daughter. This involves offering lengthy critiques of me *to me.*

A good girl. Had loads of potential but messed it all up. And she's putting on weight now too, probably all that wine she drinks. I'd have liked a grandchild, but it didn't suit her.

I preferred her nostalgic and crying for the sea.

***

I have not yet decided if I will meet Piotr. I'm already running through how our evening might play out. We will go out. Italian. Nothing too expensive. Between the antipasti and secondi, he'll say that Donald Trump was not that bad, and I will dismiss the idea of dessert, even if the tiramisu in this backstreet place with its laminated menus is said to be legendary.

Or it could be one of those rare, rare nights when everything has lined up. Every joke lands, we like all the same things and more than anything, I feel that chemical fizz, knowing that in a couple of hours, I will kiss him, or he will kiss me. Then, we'll test the shape of this thing, try to find a way to interlock and not destroy the other's orbit. I will tell my mother then, that the thing she has always wanted for me has happened, before her brain finally sinks into the swamp.

Rarely are things so clearly cut. Instead, Piotr and I will get on reasonably well, enough for it to be enough for now. There will be three dates, maybe four, some decent sex. It will fizzle out in weeks. We'll have our stories ready to swap. I'll tell him my mother has to be the focus of my life. He will say that work is demanding and he's moving to nightshifts, which he may or may not have actually requested.

In the days where my mother is actively dying, I will be at the hospital all the time, holding a tiny pink sponge on a stick up to her parched, puckered mouth. I will watch her lungs heaving and heaving as if she is lost at sea, grasping at the sky before the next wave comes. I will see Piotr at the vending machine, buying energy drinks, in green or orange, to get through the nightshift. I'll keep buying the pink-wrapper bar that she's long past eating. We will be polite. He'll ask after her and we'll part. Me heading for a walk, a break from the airless ward, the HESPIS radiator, the sense that soon, my mother won't be here.

And then, one final day I will exit these same doors and she will no longer be in the world. The addicts will still be squabbling outside the shop across the road, men loitering by the bookies will suck deeply on their cigarettes. Dubhín will be waiting for me in the window, and later we'll walk along the canal, watching the sky turn from pink to navy, the promise of a new year not far away.

Sound Distraction

Anna Jean Hughes

Present

I am not asleep. There is something in the stark mid-dark. I sit, up into the night, and watch as the pitch slit behind the door grows open. My mouth is full of heart, but it's only Pearl stretching herself through the gap. She stands, soldier-like, hands bunched beautiful at her sides. She won't catch my eye, just stares at my nan's quilt. Nanny Ann. Some woman she was. Some pig. I try to remember the last time this notquite girl tried to crawl into my bed, there's a pattern to it, but I can't make the memories line up.

'Did you have a sad dream?'

I never say bad because it's not the dream's fault.

'It was horrible, Mams,' and she branches for me as a tree would, hair in a fuss about her face. 'I was at our place, sitting underneath the laurel tree in the garden with Dad, but his face wasn't there.'

Our place gone.

I step onto the rag rug, letting my toes root down into the fabric of life before she was born. I made it when I was fat-full of her, stripping the dresses that I figured would never again fit a body so brimming with baby.

'No eyes, no mouth, just this seething nothing.'

'Pearl?'

But she's still there, seeing him. It's writ all over her face – her dad yawning his death at our big little girl. I touch her hand. She has beautiful hands; fingers tapered and long, like a ballet. Touch her wrist. Bringing her down to me and the real.

After Bobby died, all we did was sleep in a heap, clutching at each other to heat the nightmare into something fit for the day.

I give her shoulder a rub and we flump into bed, tucking into one another, like holding an egg in my hand, even though she's too old to be hodgehegging into bed with me. I can feel the lace of the nightmare on her, caught on the hedge of her shoulders as she sinks into the mattress.

'Sqwanch up, Peep, you're letting all the cold in.'

And I hate him. Let me for a minute. Years gone by, lost in a life, and none of it getting better. Never easier. The pressure to live for her. Harder and harder and I squeeze this daughter of ours hard. So hard she makes that growling noise, like an old teddy bear turned upside down. Her scalp smells of Bobby – bonfires in the life of summer. I pang, filled to the pores with missing.

She weeps into his pillow, the one I embroidered with his initials – B.S. Made him laugh every time he butted heads with it at night. O.D. Total BS.

'You and me, Peep. It's you and me now.'

On a sigh she says a little word, 'Umami.'

And this is what Bobby called us, the three of us – You, Ma and Me.

Her breath is longer as her sadness slows. I quieten my own to match hers, but I won't go under again, not with Pearl's grief squatting on my breast.

His guitar winks at me from the corner of the room.

I am in the wrong shop. I want to get Pearl something, because of starting at sixth-form college, and it has to be new. Not the usual clobber from the Mind. I don't want her being chased by the ghosts of past owners at the big school. No one wants to be haunted by a tweed jacket. Yet this place is a temple built to sexup kids. The thing I have in my hand has a frou-frou skirt covered in tiny horses the colour of a toxic rainbow.

Sparkle pony. She used to have one and all, Pearl; brought to her seventh birthday party by her best friend so I'd no time to doctor the present. Always had to watch that Andrea. Dre. It was purple and my girl loved it so much that it lost the scratch and sniff smell it had on its blueberry arse.

I go to put the dress back and see a woman staring at me in the trying place. And I'm trying to place her too. She's familiar, though everyone is when you work down the pub. Occupational tabard. But she's squinty at me and so I turn and march right out those shifty doors with the fucking dress still in my hands and there's such a noise. I run back in, but the moment I do, I'm clapped by some guy.

'Come on, Glady. What you playing at?'

'Oh hello, love. Look, I'm innocent. I wouldn't steal', I hold it out from me and it streams from my hand in a sneer, 'this.'

He just gives me a crossword grin and takes it, then walks it to the pole I'd nicked it off and gently slides it back in. I like his kindness with this little pony frock, he treats it ever so nice and when he turns to me, he's all twinkly.

'You working the Shillelagh on Friday?'

'Always do, big man.'

And I only call him that because that's what he is, but I can see he's happy with it. I've no idea of his name. I call everyone something else because names have never been my thing. Ronnie is the only person who gets his given in the pub. And nothing else. I called him Ronald once, only because he was being a spoon, and he made me clean the toilets every shift for a month.

He's staring at me now, the man, and I have a slippery feeling that I've said something out loud while thinking about cleaning Ronald's toilets.

'What is it?'

'You should come for a drink with me.'

'Should I? But I don't. Drink, I mean,' because that was Bobby's thing. Drunk.

'Coffee then, isn't that what young people do when off a courting, drink coffee?'

A courting he says. And he twinkles at me all over again and years gone by. Cold in a bed and him old in the ground.

'I do drink coffee.'

'You ever noticed your pee sparkle in the loo?'

And I'm saying this stupid thing to stop myself blurting about the new man. Though it was sparkling this morning. It's all that coffee.

'You're so weird.'

'No, I know, but also, I had one of those vitamin bath bombs you gave me and so it was radioactive sparkle. Honestly like that glitter powder you put on your eyes. But in the loo.' Inside I'm smiling so. New woman.

Pearl is peering at me, her little nose holes flaring slightly and a half-cut smile on her face.

'Have you taken something?'

'Taken something like what?'

'You know like what.'

Prune.

'No, I have not. It's,' and I squint at the clock on the wall, but he won't tell me nothing, 'daylight. And a Wednesday.' And I close my arms in affront.

'It's Friday, Mams.' She brings me in for a tight squeeze and I like it. She's younger since he died but cuddling her tight always makes me feel at home. She lets me go and makes for the door with a, 'Get off to Ronnie and don't tell anyone at the Shillelagh about your sparkling pee.'

Where does she go to in such a flush?

The Shillelagh is a gobby place, huffing at me with its yeasty breath as I step through the thick red of the door. Pocket money, Bobby said. I was only twiddling my hands into butter at home, with Pearl at school and no records to press. But these pocket pennies fast became living money. There's no bank for ageing mock-stars.

Ronnie's eyes when he sees me are a picture of stealth. They're stuck to me all the way from the door to the bar.

'What's it now, Ronnie?'

'You're ninety minutes late.'

'I am not, I came straight here.'

And here is only over the hill from there. I don't bother looking at the clock, because he's always lying, but the numbers on my phone do seem to spell an after.

'This is your first warning, Glady.'

I hum one of mine and Bobby's songs at him, then run through the swing door to the back and into the hot wine steam coming off the glass cleaner. I was shucking the beards off oysters the summer I was Pearl's age. The only thing she shucks is her phone, such a waste of face.

I get myself behind the shiny taps and who'd I see but – there's a pop in my throat and I smile so big and wide it makes my teeth hurt. It's not though. Bobby. When he turns his face to me I see it is only, 'Hello big man. What are you drinking?'

'Glad tidings indeed.'

The giggle that comes out of me is not becoming. I can see so on Ronnie's face.

'Well?'

'Pint of Guinness, and one for yourself.'

'I don't though.'

But perhaps I do. Just the once.

I haven't been this drunk since Bobby did what he did. Don't really. Drink. He drank for two, and here I am winking into a bottleneck to see what it's saying, but it just gasps its breath at me. Whine. There's another one in the fridge, ready to talk, but when I pick up the twirly-armed thing Pearl raises an eye and then gets her head back down to flick at her screen some more. She's fierce at me.

I unwind the cork from the twizzle for something to do.

'You know,' but I've no idea what's about to come out my mouth till it does, here goes: 'when I was young, my favourite thing was to get your dad to lie on me.' And I did. Loved that – the weight of him. My brilliant man. I peek at Pearl through my hair, and she grins at the table, then clatters her phone down and gets that fog on her she always gets when I talk about him.

'In a sexy way?'

'No,' and I chuck the cork in her general direction. 'I just liked the pressure of him on me.'

'Ick,' but she's smiling fit to break her face. 'I wonder,' says Pearl, then stops. I want to chivvy her along, fill in the blanks. But I know this only makes her oyster up.

And I find myself wondering myself, if she has had sexy ways.

'What about this one?' she's messing with her food.

'This what?'

Pearl casts a glance, fly fishing, and then stands up to put her plate in the sink, with its full half of half a whole lasagne on there. Posh shop lasagne. Cost the same as you'd get in the caff on the high street. I pick a clementine out of the bowl and concentrate on that.

'Oh him.'

'Yes him.'

I hold a segment up to the light, checking it for pips and then hand it to Pearl.

'He has curly hair.'

'You met him at the Shillelagh?'

'I did.' Best not tell her I met him shoplifting.

'Does that make him an Irishman?'

'Drinking in an Irish pub does not make him Irish.'

'Round here it does.' She's about to turn the water on the lasagne, to wash it all down the hole, but I frog up and take the plate off her, scraping it, peas and all, into an old margarine tub that sits in wait. 'That's breakfast right there. Wasteful harpy.'

But her face is scrunched as a horoscope. She's braving something and it's got to be Bobby. Our umami. Such a flavour. Decades with it and years without, years with no one else. This big man, he'll do for now. Hell, he does do too. It, I mean. He's not for us though, never for here. For her.

'It's not like you'll meet him, Peep. He'll not be coming to our place, that's a promise.'

I watch the fret slide from her face and wipe my hands to give her a cuddle.

'Have you seen my baccie?'

'It was over by the breadbox last I saw.'

It was there, fat like a rabbit behind my blue and white enamel box. With its *Bread* written in movie-star font.

In the time it took me to roll my fag, Pearl has cleared the wet plates onto the sideboard, good girl, and is looking like bedtime.

'The night is adolescent, darling.' I say it in my Queenie voice. She snorts at that. 'Will you stay till I finish this?'

'I have orientation tomorrow, Mams. I just want to lie in bed and read my phone.'

'Sure sure, love you Peep.' But I know it's because she doesn't like me drunk. Bobbing along, you'll turn up dead. Bobbydazzler.

Soon as she's up the stairs, I'm on to him. 'You up?' I ask. Though he's not a man to go to bed at nine. 'Will you come over?' Though I say it coy-carp and calm, he is not a man to be pushed. Come? Knowledge is power with this one. France is bacon! Though I know this already. Easy know. As long as Pearl never knows.

There's ash all over the table before I realise I've smoked my fag. Lasagne still on the side there. It'll spoil if it doesn't go in the fridge.

Presence

The morning is nickel plated through my curtains. Bobby would like that line. Not silvery. The light all dead and new. Someone knew. Now I know. The cloth downstairs, I left it in the sink. It'll be nasty, wiping that slick sick smell on whatever it touches.

Something big moves next to me. The mattress shifts and my body goes stiff as a tank. There was a fat cat I had that would paw at the mattress and I huff his name from under my teeth, 'Marbles?'

That cat died years ago.

Someone chucks a laugh at me and I feel the hair down my back fizz cold.

'Marbles!'

And it's him, the man that I plundered from the pub. My man. He smells of dust and Virginia smoke and rolls the thinnest fags a finger could wrangle.

'Glady, would you ever budge up and feed me some of that blanket. I've a builder's bum in bed.'

I love his round belly and the soft fat springs on it. I smooth one round my fingers like a baby snake. She had one of them once, Pearl. I got the box for it from some bloke in the Shillelagh, and a water bottle blanket. For the snake. The beard on him. Because they have no heat of their own. Not like him there, in my bed. Radiatoring. I bounce his springs and then cover him up to the neck with Nan's quilt. He's back asleep, I can see his eyebrows bugging at whatever's inside his head.

I want to wake him, to taste him again, but I want my teeth squeaky first. I often spend a morning mourning a fresh mouth.

The timer's off, my breath is in front of me, but I paid the bill this month, didn't I? Did. Toe-tipped. Pearl's door's open, not in her bed. That means she's been up to no good again. Fifteen and already. Or not.

Down the Half Moon, they should watch it, serving the young ones. They'll only get Bill on their neck. Knew a lad there a few years back, plucked himself a girl and made good with her in the car park. He being eighteen he assumed she was too, no bad assumption to make. Only to find her parents trying to send him down for statutory. Snitched up.

Wouldn't find me serving no age under eighteen. Not even my Pearl.

Am I downstairs to brush my teeth?

Someone's left the margarine out. It'll be runny like honey now.

There's a wine bullet. Did I drink with him upstairs? My mouth tastes of yes, but I clear it away now before the creep back upstairs. Silly to think that I don't want him to know I'm getting ready for him again, but I don't. Fourth time's a charm and here he's in my bed, novelty of that hasn't rubbed in yet. Pearl can't know. No.

There's a shriek and it makes all the ends of me hum. I trill up the stairs, turning too sharp on the landing and clocking my hip on the banister. It feels like a bruise.

In the door of the John is the fella, bald bum out and poor Pearl sat so small on the toilet.

'What the fuck are you doing in here?'

And he looks to me, 'Jesus, Glady.' But then turns back, stupid. 'You said it'd be all right to come back here.'

'No,' blazes Pearl. 'She never!' She lobs something at him hard, but it misses.

I shout, 'Out,' and pull at his fluffy shoulders, but he makes no move.

Pearl has a face on her like a cat and screams at him then, and at me next, 'Gladys,' and it's only ever that name in anger. 'You promised me.'

Glad Eyes.

Then the slammed door muffles the rest, though she doesn't stop her noise till I get him in my room and bang my own door. He saw my smile. I hadn't managed to shut it down in time and he had one of his own.

'It's not funny, big man.'

'No.'

'Girls need their privacy, this does not mean looking at their privates.'

'I never did.'

'What were you gawping there for?'

His hands around my face then, 'Sorry Gladrag.' And he picks me up in arms thick with strength and hoists me on to the bed.

'I haven't forgotten.'

He says, 'I know.' And he leans me back into the mattress and opens up the button on my bed shirt, kissing the skin waiting there. And Pearl only down the corridor.

'I never forget.'

'So I hear,' and he undoes another button. It makes my chest hold tight when he kisses me again.

Abstemious.

'Don't you forget it.'

Steamy.

'I won't,' and he takes my nipple in his mouth. I think of what it must look like, wet crêpe. I think of his tongue on me and stopper myself from making a sound. I can hear the clitter-clatter of my hard-footed girl as she brats her way to her room. The wood on wood. I think of the trouble I'll be in and beam, giving in to this man between my legs. He skins my bed shirt from me and it splays its plaid wings.

My teeth are still murky.

Pearl's reading at something pinned up and does it loud when she sees me, '*If I should die before I wake, then do these things, for fuck sake.*' She sets her face in a cross and puts her hand on her hip. 'It doesn't scan, this.'

'Yes, thank you, Peep.'

'There should be an apostrophe *s* after the fuck and all.'

'And here's me thinking I'm the lyricist.'

She's older today than she was before, grown in the face.

'What's this about, Mams?'

I try to take a good look at it, but she stands in the way, so I turn and make like it's nothing. 'Where's my baccie gone to now?'

'It's by the door on the radiator.'

And off I go to get it and it's all clammy and deflated. The warm's not on.

'Here it is.' I run down the corridor and bop her on the nose with it.

'You let that man in the house.'

'He's gone now.'

'He was here again?'

I sidle back, casual as a cucumber, and owl at the flap of paper. A list of house to-dos and I must've written them down in the giblet hours when sleep wouldn't come. 'I was thinking how lost you'd be is all. If you didn't know you had to mop up the juice from under the chilly drawers every week. The thing would flood the kitchen. Will somebody please think of the carrots!'

'Where would I be without you and your lists?'

'Listless, Peep. That's where you'd be.'

That got a smile from her. What a smile.

'Honestly, Mams, I'm fine. You're fine. We're fine.'

I look about her for something distracting and there's my margarine out on the side, I budge her away and put it in the cold cupboard, but she's still on the sore path.

'He looks like an overgrown cherub. What's the attraction?'

Skin on skin is what it is. He has lit something up, this man with the curds of curls across his chest. Even the smell of him is a taste I have inside me.

'Why'd you let him in the house, Mams?'

'He's just a bit of fun, Pearl.'

I've been sitting here, coming down and getting up to her room. She's gone. Razzle dazzle. And wasn't I the same? I was, toe-tipping out the walldoor, not proper, skittling down the old tree to freedom. I drink at the cup in front of me, but the tea is long cold in my hand. Makes good pastry. We have a deal, me and Pearl, and it's a good one – she comes home and I don't worry. The point is, there is a point. The point is she's only little. Little Peep. And I'm doing the thing we promised we wouldn't, Bobby and me, sitting up and fretting all bourgeoisie, as a mum would. I'm not mumsy. Mamsy. I stand and feel a hot trash of rage, take the stairs like they owe me something and racket at her door, throw it open, but she's not there. She's gone.

Downstairs I have another sip of the drink in my hand, but the wine is long warm. I ask the time, but he's keeping his hands to himself. That girl has been out all night, up to what knows who. And I've been go-going up and down to her room so much that I'm too angry now. Can't sleep when she won't sleep.

I drag myself up the stairs and bust in through the door only to find her in a jolt in bed.

'What's up, Mams? Are you okay?'

But she's up to something and I pull the handle hard, just to hear the slam.

Sitting at the table in the dark I look about me and I'm gasping. It hurts to catch my breath, I'm trying to net it with my lungs, but it fights at me and I'm overcome. My head is cobwebbed. I rest my face hard on my hands and try not to think of it, try not to imagine the world in which Pearl lives alone. I fling my hands out and an empty bottle bowls to the floor and sings in a spin. I put it away. Just another thing for Pearl to see. She's seen too much; those endless mornings after Bobby's nights before. My little Peep. I go upstairs, just to check, to see on her, feeling that wing of panic I used to get when she was nothing but a midge in her cot.

Inside the room is curdled with dreams and I can smell Pearl's breath. I go in slinky and sit on her bed, stroke her hair and sigh my love into her ear.

'Where have you been, girl?'

'I was just at college.'

But her face is a slantwise and I can see she's keeping something for herself.

'What, all the day?'

'Yes, you dweeb, "all the day".'

'Dweeb?'

She rolls those blinkers any harder they're going to plop out on their stalks. She's up to no good, I can tell. I was the same, skulking along the silent night of a sleeping house, riding the throb of escape.

'Were you out with that Dre last night?'

'Why do you say it like that? You've known her long as you've known me.'

'She's a fast one.'

'I don't even know what that's supposed to mean. Is there food?' and she clatters at the white door so hard the door's fit to come off its pegs.

'There's that lasagne left over from the other night?'

'What lasagne?'

I crinkle my face trying to think of when and start to hunt about the place, opening and flapping doors.

'Would it not be in the fridge?'

'Hmmm?'

But Pearl has found a little box under the sink and is peeling at the lid. It comes off with pop. Her tongue's out and complaining before I see what she's getting at.

'Fucking hell, it's grown teeth.'

My funny girl, Pearl.

Inside is a face of rot.

'How long's this been here?'

'What is it?'

'I'm guessing lasagne.' She waggles it at me; little beads move back and forth.

'And what are those?'

'Peas. Jesus, what's with you?'

'Nothing that a fag won't fix.' But as I look about for my pouch there's a tremor in my thighs and I know that it's going to take more than fags to fix this.

'Your baccie's on the chair in the lounge.'

I make my way there on broomstick legs, only to hear her chuntering away about food again. Then there's a gap in the talking. Whatever happened to that snake?

I'm rolling a cigarette.

'Wait, is this the lasagne from September?' she shouts.

'What's that?'

She's followed me into the comfy room.

'This,' and there's the butter box again. 'Is it from my first week at college?'

'I don't know what that is.'

'But that was two months ago. And why all the empty wine bottles under the sink?'

Her face is goggled and a thing crops into my head from the after school fun club I did when I was a titch, 'What a to-do to die today, at a minute or two to two. A thing distinctly hard to say, but harder still to do. And a dragon will come when he hears the drum. At a minute or two to two today, at a minute or two to two.' I look over at her, busting with grins, but she goggles some more, 'It's ten past six, Mams.'

'That wasn't me time-telling, Pearl. Let's call in a take a break. I can't be doing with this.'

'Wait, haven't you got a shift? It's Friday.'

Is it? My fingers are tight on the sticky fag paper.

'How would I know it's Friday? What does it smell like?'

'You should go, Mams. Ronnie's going to be pissed. He told you last week that you're on final warning.'

'Ronnie can go fuck spiders.'

'I'm not sure he could, even if he wanted to.'

And that is so funny I need a pee, to see some sparkle, and I run upstairs to the toilet before it catches me out.

'I'm off to Dre's for tea,' she shouts up at me. 'Go to work.'

The door bangs and I stand up and pull up my kegs, only they're a bit squelchy. So, I head into my room to change into new ones. My hands wrap around the throat of Bobby's guitar, it's up for a thrum and I sit down on the edge of the bed.

Knock knock. Halted breath, but there's nothing. Woken by something. The scrinch of Pearl's door catching. Learnt to hate that music, metal kissing metal in the dark. Still drunk on sleep. The after times in the pub, too long locked in. Old Nanny Ann watching Pearl at night. Batwing. Always dreaming on the settee when we come in from the night.

'Who's there?'

Some watchdog. Watch bitch.

Tick tock. Heating down.

There goes the scrinch again. She's up to no good.

My feet aren't at the foot of the bed and so it's tiptoes to Pearl's room. With an ear pressed heavy on her door, I can hear the wood breathe, but it's shut fast and she sleeps light that one. A shiver takes hold. I look to the gloom for hints. It is the witchy hour and the only thing that'll protect me now is Nan's quilt.

Ticktocktick.

The house is upset and I'm panting like a fox, prickled with fear. Danger is when there's only one. I am standing alone in the dark with nothing on my feet.

Someone is here.

Tockticktock.

That clocking off, it's so loud.

Take the stairs on, two feet at a time. Down. Step together. Next. Step together. If I take long enough will it be gone by the bottom?

Humming now. A man voice. In the room with the humming cupboard.

Cold riddles all along me.

The corridor worms away like a sand river. There is someone at the end of it.

'Get out!'

'Gladrag?'

Who would use that name? And there he is, stepping onto my shadow.

'What are you doing here?'

'You called me over, babe.'

'I never, at this time.'

'No, before. Anyway,' and he leans his bristles towards me then past. 'Got to run. See you again, yeah?'

Ticktocktick.

I turn.

'Sorry,' he says, handing me the tick tock from the upright. 'I messed with it and couldn't get it to turn off. What even is it anyway?'

Tick tock but doesn't tell the time.

I glare at the thing, heavy in my hand, made of trees with its seesawing face and I look up at the man to tell him No, I don't know. But it is light in the door glass, and he's gone. It's just me in my cold feet, counting away a beat.

'What do you have against the lady doctor?'

'I don't, love.'

'You do, what is it?'

'She's the sort that eats her pizza with a knife and spoon.'

Pearl puffs, 'Who would do that?'

And spoon wasn't right. Not spooning. Pizza with a spoon?

'Exactly.'

'But no one does that, Mams. You're not making sense.'

'Exactly.'

Easier to leave this one be. Bye the by.

'Mams?'

'You seen my baccie?'

'It's on the table.'

But it's not and my fingers itch to feel the plump of it. 'Where Peep?'

'Right there, in front of you,' and she lobs something into my lap. It's soft and with ears, a bunnykin, fur like a lucky footring.

'What's this?' I hold it up to Pearl, the head of it flopping deadly over my fingers. And when I look into her sad I want to take all the words back into my mouth and swallow them.

There's a line of teeth halving its pouchy belly. I pull at a tag and the teeth shout open wide and there are the sticky papers and my shreds to put in them.

It is called a metronome.

The box is on and shouting at me.

'Something's not right, Mams.'

To never be lonely again, Bobby said. I have to live. Discombobbylating.

'I found this under the sink again.'

She stretches a little garden at me, there's grass in there, a rolling hill. It looks like a graveyard.

'That's so pretty. Did you make it?'

Peep shuts her face and her shoulders heave up. Fall down. She puts the little garden on the fluffy floor and puts her head on the flat of my legs.

'What is wrong with you?' Muffling.

She's making me all damp with her eyes. Pulling at me. Pulling. She pulls.

'Mams, I want you back. Come back.'

Where do I go though? Where does she think I've been? Right here is where.

Presented

The sight of gloom in the looking glass gives my skin a tickle. Fear left-rights over each arm curl in turn, till I'm sprung. I close myself and then dare another look – mouth side open and eyes wide. I close myself.

The thing I'm in is jabbing at me, makes me sit like manners, and there's nowhere for my hands but all over themselves. I stare into them so I don't see the looking glass. Here's the church and there's the steeple, open the door and see all the –

Peep.

She'd better be in her bed.

The door handle feels strange in my hand, long and cold instead of round and warm. My hand feels slick on it, and it slips off with a slang.

'Pearl?'

The night whispers back at me. This is not my room.

'Dad killed himself in a laurel bush.'

I look. The woman that is always here is not looking at me. Her face lines are high.

'She says this a lot, I wondered if it was something real?'

'It's real. He did – hanged himself when she was seventeen.'

He did, did he?

'Poor thing.'

And her big face moon is in mine.

'You poor thing. What can that have been like?'

Where's my baccie?

'Her fingers keep doing that, it's like she's warming the tips of them.'

'She's rolling herself a cigarette.'

'Oh, well there's no smoking allowed in here. That wouldn't do at all.'

'Where's the harm?'

'Young lady, it's probably all that poison that got your poor mother in this disastrous state. Anyway, I'll leave you two alone. Just shout if you need anything, okay? Toodaloo.' Waggling.

Ridiculous creature.

And then there's she. She's started mid. I've missed the start.

'I've been staying with Dre, while social services work out what to do with me.'

Never liked that one. Makes her head all colours. Brassy.

She holds something out to me. It's orange round. Only small. I don't take it, so she starts to tear its skirt off. Underneath it's all bare and white. I think of it in my mouth, and it fills. We had them, little things in a plank square, Santa-time; they came to the door wrapped in crinkles.

'Ronnie gave me your last pay check in cash and he's worked out how to get your disability to me too. It's only going to last six months though, from when you were admitted.'

The orange is on the floor in bits.

Like at the flickies? I eyeball about me. No flickies here.

194

'He was saying I could take some shifts in the kitchen if I need. But I can't do bar till I'm eighteen.'

And the salt of it. Shucks.

The girl puts a thick orange smile in my hand and I hold it up to the light, but I don't know why.

'The council came and took the house, Mams. I didn't know what to do with all our stuff, so Ronnie's stashed it in that room above the Shillelagh for now. He's been so good to us.'

That moustache being nice is he. Someone's taken all the paint off my finger hards. They're naked. I hold them up to show the girl, maybe she's here to do that. But her big balls are swimming in oceans.

'Mams, where did you go?'

It's my Pearl.

'I'm here, girl.'

And there's a word hot in the place where the loud goes, 'Umami'. She clings till it hurts, at where my warm thing meets my head. 'Don't go. Please.'

I touch my face and the fingers come off all wet.

Where am I going to?

I'm right here.

Coming and Going

Paul McVeigh

'Alright, son?' Dad says, his words sounding soft like he's chewed them.

It's taken me by surprise, the 'son', as Dad has been completely absent for the last few weeks. Usually, it's a case of coming and going. The going has been taking longer and the coming shorter. Recently, someone's been there, just not the man who was my dad. A new man who bore no resemblance to the Dad I knew, physically or in personality. My not-dad. I'm coming to terms with the fact that one day he will be gone forever, while to some it will look like he's still right here with us.

I roll with his return and see just how far we can go with it before it loses momentum. I still don't know what this version of Dad remembers or how long before some other version takes his place.

'Alright, Dad,' I smile, keeping the energy high. 'How are you feeling today?'

'Good-good,' he says, rubbing his hands the way he used to when he got excited. This is a good day. 'Where's Lee-anne?'

It takes a second for me to adjust. So, we're within a three-year period, around fifteen years ago. We've been told not to challenge him, not to force him into the present as it can be confusing and even traumatic. So, for now, I'm straight. I go back into the closet.

'Lee-anne's away with work, Dad,' I say, moving people and places from the past around in my head. I try to suppress the stench of stale emotions, the shifting of mental furniture he has uncovered. At the same time, I'm inventing a present-day story that fits with the history. These are the kind of mental gymnastics I'm well prepared for after having to hide my sexuality for all those years. Years of being forced to lie, spinning so many alternate realities and it became impossible to keep all the plates balancing on their ridiculously thin sticks.

'Sure, what about the wedding?' Dad's eyes fix on a place in mid-air.

My eyes join his, staring into the same space, as if the past existed there and was playing out right in front of us. I think about that time. It could have gone so badly – for me and her and the families. Although cancelling was awful, and bad enough, at least I stopped it before I went through with the wedding. I couldn't do that to her. I did love her, but I knew something was missing and I couldn't deny her the chance to have it all.

'You're not having trouble are you?' Dad says, bringing me back. 'You have to get all that business sorted before, you know.' He raises his eyebrows.

'No,' I say, 'All's going well. She's off seeing the priest, about all that.'

'Do you not have to be there with her?' Dad looks at me from the corners of his eyes. If I didn't know better, I'd say he was trying catch me out in a lie. Leading a double life all those years definitely took a toll on our relationship, preventing us from getting close. I think he was always trying to work me out.

'No, the priest needs to go through the process with her, alone, about the conversion,' I say. 'Between her and the Big Man and all that.'

'What conversion?' Dad looks totally confused.

I thought that was what he was talking about. For us to get married in the church I'd grown up in Lee-anne had to convert to Catholicism. I need to be careful what I say. Anything confusing or contentious can set him off. He's always been formidable, but this disease, if that's what it is, has made him violent at times.

'I mean about the arrangements, the rehearsal, the flowers and what have you,' he says.

'Ach, no, best leave her to it,' I say. 'Sure, what use would I be with all that stuff?'

I've never been that 'bloke', but it's always been easier with Dad to pretend that I was the man he wanted me to be. To be fair, it wasn't just him. Back then, it seemed like the whole world wanted me to be someone else and it was more exhausting and dangerous fighting against that than it was pretending to be straight. Though before I came out, before his illness, there'd be, at times, a pause from Dad after my performance as the macho Irish male. Then his silence would say everything we'd been avoiding for years.

Dad settles into his chair, nestles his head into the red tartan blanket folded over the back, and closes his eyes. The blanket came along with the National Trust membership I got when we started to lose him. I'd take him out to country piles and gardens at the weekends where we'd walk and talk a little and have tea and cake in fusty cafés. When the weather allowed, he liked to sit in the grounds of these old places. He'd wrap the blanket around his legs and make jokes about how grand it was to be chauffeured about to check on his estates.

Dad's mouth drops open as he falls asleep and the snores come from the back of his throat. His lips are dry and cracked, I'll remind the nurses – if they are actually nurses; half of them look like they are on work experience from school. Dad's cheeks are sunken as if invisible weights sit on them. It's even more pronounced when he sleeps with his head tilted back. They took out all of his teeth. They gave their reasons, but I knew the real reason why: they weren't brushing his teeth so they rotted. Ok, I know it can't have been easy looking after him but removing his teeth means he can only eat soft food and drink liquid meals. He looks so much older now. It's changed the shape of his face so dramatically you'd barely recognise him from before. Though I feel terrible for thinking it, when his face is relaxed and his cheeks sink in, he reminds of me of the painting *The Scream*. It's very unsettling. I understand why Teresa has stopped bringing her kids. They got so upset. Teresa only comes on special occasions now herself.

I shake my head and rub my face to get rid of the image. I take a slow, deep breath and try to relax. I scan the room for distraction. A wife is giving a hand massage. A daughter is brushing long, pale-yellow hair. A grandchild pokes a colostomy bag with his finger. A son-in-law is tapping his phone while his leg bounces from boredom.

The largest wall in this oddly shaped room is floor-to-ceiling glass. The main window, in the centre, is cracked on the bottom-right corner. A square of gauze provides a temporary plaster on the wound. Outside, on the ground below, the burnt carcass of the bonfire remains. I heard that the residents had been brought to the window to watch the local housing estate's annual July Twelfth 'celebrations'. Many of the elderly Protestants would have remembered the annual eleventh-night festivities – burning bonfires with Irish flags and effigies of Catholics. Even the extreme heat cracking the window hadn't bothered the patients, the nurse said. Apparently Dad loved it, had an absolute ball. God, if Dad – my before dad – could look at himself now, he'd be beyond mortified. It seems as if no thought was given to those who might have terrible memories of bonfire night. But if Dad had a ball, I suppose there's no point in getting annoyed on principle alone. Though being Northern Irish I feel genetically compelled to.

The cracked window though? I feel like I should complain about that. Who exactly would I complain to? And was it really the dementia home's fault? And if I did complain, would the nurses treat Dad differently when I left him in their care? You hear such horror stories. There was that poor woman from Ardoyne, Julie something, my friend went to school with her daughter and heard it directly from the family. Julie had been a walker. One of those whose dementia wouldn't let them sit still. She'd spent the day walking along the corridors of her rest home until she hit a locked door, turn around, and walk back again. Coming and going, Julie would say 'hello' each time she passed anyone. And everyone loved her, my friend said. Always smiling. Always waving. One morning, the family got an urgent call to get down to the home. No one knew how it had happened. Or who did it. Another patient, they guessed. But, the family said, for all they knew it could have been a member of staff. A purple, swollen eye and bruises all over her body. And a silence of unspeakable things that had been done to her.

Dad was in a care home in a Catholic area but we moved him after he had a bad fall. Now I can see how it could have happened on anyone's watch. Dad had begun to deteriorate. At the time, we didn't want to admit it, and who knew if it was a fall, right? We just didn't want to take any chances.

For the most part the whole Catholic/Protestant thing doesn't come into the home once you're inside and away from the flags and wall 'art' on the streets. There's the odd tattoo on a helper's arm, the occasional snippet of conversation floating about when staff are chatting with their tea. This has taken it to a whole new level though. Watching a bonfire. A bonfire that has damaged the building and no one seems to bat an eye.

Dad's eyes open. 'Are you still here?'

'I've not been here that long,' I answer.

'How long was I asleep?'

'Just a few minutes.'

'Where's John?'

My face relaxes, telling me that it must have been stressed. 'John's at work.'

'Hard worker, that fella. You did well there.'

'I know it.'

'When they letting me go home?' Dad presses his hands down on the arms of the chair to push himself up.

'Well, they're still waiting on the results of your tests.' I press my hand down firmly on one of his arms and Dad looks at it. 'Once we get those, you'll be straight home.' He sits back in slow motion. Lying to Dad comes easily to me after all the years of practice.

There is no home any longer. Dad's house was sold to cover old tax bills and the cost of care. Who knew it would be so expensive? And the mess of Dad's affairs. There were letters unopened in a drawer in the kitchen, under the cushions on the sofa, in the bread bin and cupboards. Fines that had grown with each unanswered warning. Tax returns not filed. He was a bit of a rebel – we were embarrassed about it as kids, impressed by it in our twenties, then finally fucked by it when he got sick. All those back taxes and old fines had to be paid from his savings and the house. His money, for sure, but so much for his promises of nest eggs for us. They were well and truly hatched. And no will. Months of going through papers that went back years. Searching through his house and emptying it before we sold it. It was like he was already dead.

I was glad Dad and I had reconciled by then. I don't know how I would have felt if we'd left it until he got sick, knowing that any chance of meaningful healing would have been lost. It's meant I could be there with him through everything. It means I can be here now.

It took me years to come out to Dad. Well, first I had to come out to myself. I knew, but I didn't want to know. I knew from the jokes that were made and the bullying that went on around me that these weren't thoughts a boy was supposed to have. And I knew that everyone despised gay people. I'd never heard one positive thing said about being gay. I knew it was against my – and seemingly, all – religious beliefs. I didn't want to consider giving up my family, friends, religion – the world as I knew it then. Besides, I was a people-pleaser. All I really wanted was to make everyone happy. I didn't want to be what seemed to be the worst thing a boy could be. It took me years to accept that there are other kinds of boys. It took even longer to accept I was one of them. I was so used to telling lies, so I could be a person people liked and loved, that I lied to myself constantly too.

When I realised that it wasn't a choice, that I was what I was, I had to grapple with how, or, indeed, if I would tell Dad. My sister told me that I had no right to tell him and Mum. That it would be selfish of me. 'Is the apology for the person receiving it or more about the person giving it needing forgiveness?' she asked. 'You're doing this for you without a thought for the pain it will cause them. Just go ahead and live your life. There's no need for them to know.'

I could see her point. What they didn't know wouldn't hurt them! I didn't want to hurt them. In fact, I'd used that excuse to myself in the years leading up this point. But, at the end of the day, I knew that, deep down, my parents knew, and they knew I knew they knew etc. ... So, why keep up the lie? It was exhausting pretending to be someone I wasn't. My parents got to be themselves, and so did my sister. She got to have her partner and family welcomed into our clan. Why not me and mine? Why did I have to always be on the outside at family gatherings? Appearing as the unloved even while I was loved. Explaining to my partner how he wasn't invited. He couldn't be invited because he didn't exist as far my parents were concerned.

In the end, I came out to Mum and Dad because I was forced to. Sam, a straight guy from work, spotted me at a gay bar. He'd been there with a gay friend, he said. Sam approached me about it one day while making coffee in the staff room. He didn't understand why I wasn't out at work. I guess he saw how uncomfortable I was with the conversation, just how much I feared coming out. He asked whether I was out to my family and I didn't think to lie. He walked off and I naively thought that was the end of it.

It started one day with something that seemed quite natural. The guys were going to the pub for a drink after work. Sam didn't have any cash on him so he asked me for a loan of a few quid. He'd give it back to me tomorrow. I didn't know him that well, so it was odd. There was a very slight smile on his face that made me know to give the money to him. He didn't give it back that time. Nor the next time, or the next.

Then he got cocky. He threatened to out me to my family unless I paid him a ridiculous amount of money. I even considered it, daft as it sounds. And here's the thing: if he hadn't been so greedy, asking for so much, I probably would have paid it. He assumed my nice accent meant I came from money when, like most of my ilk trying to make it in middle-class professions, I had softened my working-class accent and kept talk about my background to a minimum.

That's when I decided to come out. I had no choice, really. It was the only way to stop this guy having power over me. So, in the end, no real integrity, none of the gay pride everyone goes on about. It was fear and desperation which forced my hand.

I took my parents to lunch in a trying-to-be-posh hotel restaurant. My stomach was in bits so I swirled my soup round and round the bowl creating a mini whirlpool, one I wished would swallow me up. Meanwhile, Mum chatted away about her grandchildren and upcoming family events. I just blurted it out. That I'd been with women and ... men. There was barely a pause before Mum asked me to pass the salt. I did. She was right. The soup wasn't salty enough. I had some too. So did Dad. Here was something we all had in common. The need for salty soup.

That was it. Sort of. When Mum went to the toilet, I told Dad that I had struggled with being honest with them. I apologised for telling them like this but explained what had happened with the guy at work. I could see the veins in his hand raise as he gripped his spoon, but he didn't say a word. We never really talked about it after that. I told the guy at work that I'd come out at home and to tell whoever he wanted. He didn't say anything to anyone, and I was never bothered by him again.

I say I never talked about it again with Dad but the Friday after I came out to him and Mum, he turned up outside work. He was there as we all left for the Friday pint. He was in a T-shirt that had *Proud Dad* on it in rainbow-coloured lettering. He looked so awkward. I hadn't even wanted to come out to the rest of them at work but I couldn't leave him hanging. I went over to him, and laughed. I didn't know what to say or do. Dad insisted on going to our works drink. He kept asking which one of them it was who'd been bothering me, but yer man had disappeared from the group en route.

After that though, Dad and I grew apart. He stood up for me when it mattered, was there if things were bad or I really needed him, but not so much when things were good. He didn't want to be part of my life. My gay life – my happiness. Not until years later. After Mum died.

I was the one without a family of my own and although unspoken, it was clear I was going to be the one to step in, step up for Dad. And doing that brought us together finally I guess; he knew he needed me. I think grief had softened him too. Or maybe it was just the advancing of dementia changing his personality, but by the time John came into my life, Dad was like a different man. He was so accepting of me and John, welcoming, in fact. And then, as if he'd been waiting for me to find someone, Dad started to let go.

One of the cleaners comes over. 'Your lift is waiting for you outside.'

'Thanks,' I say.

'Quite the looker,' she says.

'Thanks,' I say again, and give her a cheeky smile.

She pauses for a second then continues round the room. There are many ways of coming out.

I kiss Dad on the forehead; something I would never have done when he was well. I wonder about the ethics of this as I take the stairs to the front door.

'How was he today?' asks John.

'Told me you're a great catch,' I smile, 'so clearly not himself.'

John laughs as we pull out of the car park. The red, white and blue bunting that had hung between the lamp posts on the street had snapped and was blowing in front of us like a kite string.

'I could grab that and make a special outfit for the Pride march,' John says.

'I'd give a hand wrapping it around your neck,' I say and John laughs. He takes his hand off the gear stick and brings the back of my hand to his lips.

My Way Home

Caleb Azumah Nelson

In the kitchen, Pops and Rodney laugh that kind of loose laughter which brings a smile to everyone close. Rodney, doubled over by the sink, holds on to the counter as if letting go would mean drowning in delight. Pops, seated at our small dining table – meant for two, often repurposed for four, well, three, nowadays – holds onto his chest, trying to contain the laughter, trying to prolong this moment of joy. It's like watching a mirror, these two versions of the same person across the room from each other.

I hover by the doorway until Rodney catches my eye.

'What did I miss?' I ask.

'Pops is being Pops. Talking about his party days.'

'Look, trouble always found me, I wasn't looking for it.'

'Sure, Pops, sure.'

Rodney signals for me to come further into the room. Pops has the chess set out, the pieces arranged neatly. He's made a move and is waiting for his opponent. We – Rodney and I – share a look, because this means Pops isn't here, he's ten years back, waiting for our mother to make the next move.

'Ife, I didn't see you come in.' He hauls himself up, careful not to knock over anything from his game and, taking my hand, pulls me in for a hug. As we separate, his eyes glimmer grey in the evening light, the trace of laughter glinting at me.

'Do you know where your mother is? When is she coming home?'

'I'm not sure,' I say.

'But it's late,' he says. His face tightens with quick worry, the fluster making its way to his limbs, the rub of his hands, the twist of his fingers.

'But lemme make you a tea while you wait for her, ok? She won't be long.'

Rodney flicks the kettle on. Pops watches as I pluck mint from its stem, from a plant he placed into the soil with his own hands, last summer. The leaves briefly swim on the surface, before, like a memory, sinking under.

'You want honey?'

He nods. Rodney flicks on the radio, murmuring something along the lines of *too quiet in here*. They're playing something smooth, some jazz which lures Pops towards tiredness, so there's no need for the usual pull and tug, no need to convince him to head towards the living room to settle into more comfortable surroundings, no need to deflect the question of Mum's return, no need to see our father's sadness when something touches him – perhaps a memory hovering at the edge of his consciousness, just out of reach, or the way the light leans through the kitchen window, falling onto my face, my own features fashioned from hers – no need for any of that, just half a cup of a sweet mint tea, the nod of Pops' head as he drifts off, the smile accompanying his brief protests of *I'm not sleeping*, Rodney helping him out of the chair, out of the room, towards slumber, towards respite, towards some rest, for him and us both.

By morning, Rodney has gone – we care for Pops in shifts, half a week on, half a week off – and Pops is back in the kitchen chair. I make us a plate of scrambled eggs each and settle in opposite him. His kufi is slightly askew and I reach up to adjust it. He closes his eyes as I do, a slight smile on his face. I gaze outside at a clear September sky, light grazing the large oak, the branches swaying in the breeze. For a moment, I am lost in its rhythm. When I look back, he's watching me watch time move.

'It's like music,' he says. I place my hand on top of his, give it a short squeeze. We sit in this space, the sounds from the world like quiet percussion.

'Alright, Pops, after breakfast, me and you.' I gesture to the chessboard. He looks from me to the pieces and back to me again, sticking a fork into his eggs. He chews slowly, thoughtfully, before speaking.

'Ife, I don't want to be rude—'

'But?'

'I have been playing this game for many years. The only person who I think could beat me is your mum.'

'Well, I'll just have to prove you wrong.'

Pops raises his eyebrows. His eggs are immediately forgotten. He leans down, forward, towards the table, as if he's going to war and surveying the best point of attack. He makes a move. I counter. He makes another, I do the same. I bait him into exposure, the way Mum taught me: a few moves later, he has nowhere to go. He settles back into his chair, defeated, less upset than in awe. He shakes his head and smiles, almost to himself, already plotting and scheming his revenge.

Later in the morning, I haul one of the thicker family albums off the shelf, the one which shows their beginning – Mum and Dad – and bring it into the kitchen. Pops was initially prescribed art therapy when he began to forget, asked to hold a pencil in a bunched fist, attempt to sketch an image they'd given him. Having never been much of a visual artist, he found the work too frustrating, found that he was losing detail with each nervous line, found that he couldn't imbue the image he was making with the emotion from the source image; because even if he couldn't always remember what he was seeing, he could still *feel* it. I could see it in the excitement which dashed across his features, settling in his eyes. So now, every day, we rifle through one of the family photo albums, these untouched archives of our lives. On bad days, it's like Pops is gazing upon the life of a stranger; on good days, he's electric, speaking of the notoriety of his three-man group, pointing to the photo of him, Uncle Jimmy and Uncle Dennis, dressed in these shimmering sweatsuits, neat afros sculpted sharp and high, on the way to a function, ready to dance until they'd sweated through their clothes. Usually, he's somewhere between, like today. Seeing the photo of Mum he took a few days after they met, he fumbles as he pulls it from the clear sleeve, holds it closer so that he might be as close as possible to what was. He might murmur, *Your mother and I,* and trail off, shaking his head, the story so infinite and endless and heartbreaking. I've heard this story many times before, from her mouth, when she was alive, and from his, in the months after she passed, in the time he was desperately trying not to forget.

He holds the photo out to me. It's Mum, wearing a dress which dances somewhere between pink and purple, a coy, cheeky smile on her face – perhaps she was still trying to work Pops out. A few days before, sometime in early 1990 – neither of them could be exact with the date – Pops was driving a train from Upminster to Wimbledon. They were close to the end of the line, and he took a little extra time for himself in the cabin, watching as people trailed out onto the platform. That's when he saw Mum, splendid in the crisp sunshine. They exchanged a quick glance and Pops had to fight the urge to leave the train and its commuters where it was, leave the cabin, go towards her. She smiled at him, briefly, before glancing away, going on towards her destination.

He thought about her all day, through the rest of his shift, and when he clocked off and bumped into Uncle Dennis, near New Cross Gate where he lived, and Uncle Dennis told him about a little get-together in the evening, he was still thinking of her, wondering who she was, where she was from, *why* she was here. This why was a source of intrigue to him – having made the journey from Ghana a few years before with his own motivations, he wondered what brought others here, to London, and so he decided, as he was pulling a comb through his soft afro, letting a tiny hoop swing from his ear, he decided if he ever were to meet her again, these were the questions he would ask first.

He was still thinking of her when, at the party, Uncle Dennis pulled him close, so as to be heard better over the music, saying his girlfriend, Lucinda, had brought one of her new friends from work, Julie, and perhaps they should be introduced. She's from Ghana too, he was saying, already on the move, and my father, still thinking about this woman from the train platform, laughed when he caught sight of Julie, and she laughed too, in that way that coincidences can be a source of joy and, neither wanting to ruin the magic of the moment, they shook hands with each other, pretended this was their first meeting. When it was just them, after the dancing and the gentle ribbing from both their friends about how cosy they looked already, Pops went to ask where she was going when he'd seen her on the train, but she cut across him.

'I'm hungry,' she said. 'And there's no food here.'

'I don't live far.'

'How far are we talking? You don't want to mess with a hungry person. The line between hunger and anger is very thin, Jeremy.'

At this, my father laughed; the seriousness of her tone coming all the way round to amusement.

'A five-minute walk. And I have food.'

They left together. The walk was short, as promised, and they climbed the stairs of the house my father lived in, a house which had been separated into several living spaces. Pops had the top floor to himself, with his own bathroom and kitchen, a small living area, but his all the same. Pops indicated she should make herself at home, before disappearing into the kitchen. He heard her put on a record – she always said it was Marvin Gaye, Pops said it was Willie Hutch – but regardless, there was music. In the kitchen, he cracked several eggs into a pan, watched them sputter and pop, flipping them briefly, carefully, so the yolk was runny but sealed in. He sliced several pieces of hard-dough bread, buttered them on both sides, let them fry in the same oil as the eggs. He brought it through to the living area and they ate quickly, hungrily, while one of those soul singers crooned.

'How far do you live?' he asked.

'Not far,' she said.

It was then Pops remembered the questions he'd wanted to ask her, but she interrupted him once more, having finished her food and spotted the chess set sat on a tiny tabletop in the corner of the room.

'You know how to play?'

'I think if you played me, you'd be in trouble.'

Pops, affronted, put down his plate and pulled the table over to where they sat. They moved down to the carpet and he set up the game, eager to play. She gestured for him to go first. He made a move. She countered. He made another, she did the same, baiting him into exposing his queen. A few moves later, there was nowhere for him to go. He placed his hands atop his head, less in despair than in awe, shaking his head, almost to himself, already plotting and scheming his revenge. They played again and again, that night, the next day, when, as promised, she returned, and the next day, in the following weeks and months and years. When they moved in together, and found themselves on separate sides of the day, Pops working the day shift, Mum working the night shift at the hospital, Pops would cook breakfast for them so Mum would be greeted with food on arrival, and before he departed, before she slept, a chess game. He got closer and closer but could never beat her.

A few days later, I'm laid out flat on my bed, the dull hum of electricity coursing through the light overhead. It's 9, maybe 10 p.m. and Pops had retired earlier than usual. Around 5 p.m., I could see him beginning to fight the urge to close his eyes, let his body go slack, slide into slumber. I'm doing the same, occupying that place between consciousness and dreams, a place where my mind wanders through memories. I'm thinking of Mum, of days when she was most sick and yet still so active, still labouring over jollof for hours, still making sure we had everything we needed, still wanting to take care of us all. If she'd not sat Rodney and I down a few years ago, to tell us she was unwell, beyond treatment at this stage, if she'd not said, 'Boys there's nothing to be done but enjoy these last days together,' there would have been no warning when she left us. We wouldn't have noticed anything wrong.

Pops on the other hand has no choice. His illness stays pressed to his chest, announces itself before he can announce himself, his agency lost somewhere in the swirl of memories he keeps trying to grasp.

This is what I'm thinking when 'My Way Home' comes up on the shuffle. Not thirty seconds have gone by before Pops bursts into my room, energy humming from him like electricity.

'That music!' He listens for a moment, but nothing slides into place. 'No, no … this is different,' he says, waving away the sound.

'Hold on,' I say. I scroll through my phone looking for the sample used in the song, Gil Scott Heron's 'Home is Where the Hatred Is', hoping this is what he heard, not recognising the music but going towards the feeling. When it does begin to play, his eyes close, not with fatigue but contentment. He begins to sway and move of his own accord, moved by something beyond the sound.

'There's a song on this album … this one, this one playing was your mother's favourite but mine is near the end.'

I scroll again, gambling on 'Peace'. Once more, movement, a sway, content.

'When your mother gets home, will you play that song for her?

'I will, Pops. I will.'

'Ok. Ok.' He sighs, pleased, a man renewed. 'I love you, Ife.'

'I love you, too, Pops.'

He smiles and shuffles away quickly. I return to dream space, replaying the memory of moments just passed, a memory I hope never to forget.

Sometimes, like today, when Rodney and I cross over shifts, and neither of us have anywhere to go, or rather, when secretly it is each other's company we want, someone who understands, who doesn't need an explanation, doesn't need to be told how taxing it can be, how heartbreaking it is to watch your own father disappear into his mind, sometimes, like today, Rodney stays for dinner, helps wash up while I coax Pops out of his chair in the kitchen, towards the living room, towards his bed, and when I return to the kitchen, Rodney has already poured a little measure of spirit into glasses, which I quickly down and pour another, clinking glasses on this second one. Today, he can see how tight my grip is on the glass; he slowly, tenderly unclenches my fingers, places the glass on the side. Pulls me in so my head rests against his chest, so we might pause for a moment. It's so quiet, but I can hear the slow thud of his heart against the walls of his chest. It's like music. We sit across from each other when we separate, the chessboard on the table between us. Rodney nods at the board. I shrug, less apathy than encouragement. He makes a move, so do I. Mum taught him how to play too, so it's three rounds of stalemates before I carve out a win.

When I knock over his queen, my brother sits back in this chair, watching me. I know there are questions we both have and this is the moment when we might ask them. I know both of us wonder when Pops began to forget; wonder what started this process, what could cause the mind to disappear itself; wonder, selfishly, if the same fate awaits us both. We've done this often, circled theories into the dead of the night, swooping down on an idea, wanting to clutch tight to anything which might explain this heartbreak. But tonight, this quiet, this peace is enough. We make do with the comfort of each other's company. And not wanting to disturb this, Rodney resets the board. We play another game, play until morning comes.

When Rodney leaves, and morning light makes a home on the walls of the kitchen, I try again with the photos. Today is a good day. With each turn of the page, Pops grazes a finger across the plastic housing the photos, putting a name to each face, often with a smile. He points to Uncle Dennis, Uncle Jimmy, Auntie Claudia, Auntie Charlotte, each name quiet, considered, like he's speaking histories with each syllable. When he arrives at the image of Mum, he stops turning. Places both palms down across the pages, trying to be as close to her as possible. His smile is slow, tender, a little mournful. He doesn't hurry away.

'This is your mother,' Pops says.

I'm surprised by this introduction, so I ask, 'What was she like?'

'This is your mother,' Pops says again. He's pointing again, excitedly, the grin taking over his face. 'Your mother and I ...' I follow this trail away, into the endlessness that was their life, their love. I follow their trail back, before his illness, before hers, to the moment a train driver met a woman's gaze, her beauty striking him like a warm summer's breeze, time stopping for them both.

He sighs. 'More time. I needed more time.'

He takes my hand and places it between the photo and his, so the image is not just something I might see but feel too. We stay like this a while, until Pops shifts his hand away, gesturing to the chessboard. I raise my eyebrows, teasing him, as if asking, you sure you want me to beat you again? He waves me away. I close the photo album and take my place opposite him. He makes a move, I counter. We take this game slowly, not wanting to disturb our quiet, not wanting to disturb our peace. When we're done, maybe I'll ask him for another game, and another. Anything to make this time stretch, anything to make this time endless.

Afterword

Jane Lugea

Dementia, in its many forms, challenges our very being. Stories explore our very being. Here, I want to reflect on what makes dementia worthy of exploring through stories, and what makes stories about dementia more than just that; I suggest that they offer a chance to interrogate what it means to be human, what we humans value, how we relate and care for one another. I'll be taking a look back at the stories included in this collection, as well as considering the several years of collaborative research that led to it. My perspective is informed by my love of language: as an academic linguist, I specialise in literary language, and how the rules of a language can be exploited, manipulated and bent by its users for creative means. But creative language is not just an aesthetic artform to be appreciated. It also disrupts our usual way of seeing things, providing an alternative lens for interrogating and understanding key challenges humans face. Dementia is one of those.

For all these reasons, I embarked on an eighteen-month research project in 2020, generously funded by the UK's Arts and Humanities Research Council. The aim of the project was to explore a particular kind of contemporary fiction – that which represents the *minds* of characters with dementia. I collected 400,000 words of such fiction and looked for patterns in the way dementia and its symptoms were represented in creative writing. Some of the findings are mentioned below. I also hypothesised that seeing the world through the eyes of characters with dementia might facilitate a better understanding and awareness of the condition in readers. This possibility was explored with my fantastic co-researchers at Queen's University Belfast, who brought their expertise in ageing societies, and in gathering public attitudes and readers' opinions: Dr Gemma Carney, Dr Paula Devine and Dr Carolina Fernández-Quintanilla. Jan Carson lent us her literary talents and community engagement experience. Together, we hosted reading groups using extracts from the fiction I had studied.

Each reading group had people with different experiences of dementia: there was a group of student social workers, a group of people of who cared for loved ones with dementia, a group from the general public, as well as a group of people living with the condition. We learnt a lot from their different responses: about how fiction relates to peoples' realities, about how it can confirm, deny or challenge perceptions. The most significant thing I learnt is that creative writing offers ways of understanding dementia that medical factsheets, media representations or casual conversations cannot. Creative writing can represent the experience of living with dementia such that readers can simulate it, better understand it and maybe even better respond to it in our daily interactions.

Dementia and the person
As Jan outlined in her introduction to this anthology, dementia is an umbrella term for several hundred conditions, all of which involve a physical deterioration of some part of the brain. Despite the fact that it is clearly a physical illness, as a society we tend to focus on the mental and behavioural

changes that occur in people living with dementia. Maybe we only believe what we can see. But this focus might also arise from the fact that those mental and behavioural changes are uncomfortable to witness for those without dementia. On a personal level, dementia can wreak havoc on a loved one's personality, changing the nature of our interactions with them, and on their memory, erasing or rewriting the relationship history we share with them. On a societal level, dementia affects aspects of our being that fast-paced, neo-liberal, Western cultures hold dear: autonomy, cognitive abilities, multi-tasking (for more on this, see Ian Maleney's *Minor Monuments*). What these personal and societal reactions to dementia have in common is a perceived decay of the *person,* i.e. that dementia has reduced, diminished or erased the 'self'. To a certain extent, the self/person is defined by other people, or relationships with other people. For several decades now, advocates for 'personhood' in dementia care have been trying to emphasise the continued existence of a person behind the dementia. Despite these efforts, many representations of dementia in popular culture and conversation continue to focus on a perceived 'loss of self', or the 'dehumanising' effect of dementia.

Narrativising dementia: a paradox
I believe stories are one way of reinstating the person in our understanding of dementia, and our societal response to it. Stories invite us to depart from our own existence for a moment, to live vicariously in another person's shoes, and understand the world from their perspective. Important strides are being made by people living with dementia who are writing their own stories – testimonies to what it is really like to experience it. Surely, there is no better way to understand the person behind the dementia. But one limitation with the autobiographical story of dementia is the impossibility of capturing the later

stages of the illness, when the person with dementia can lose the ability to tell their story.

Writers of fiction are increasingly tackling dementia in their stories. I believe that there are two main reasons for this. First, the rise in literary representations of dementia is in response to an increasing societal awareness of the disease. Ageing populations and more diagnoses are resulting in a greater prevalence of the condition, so more of us are affected. As I described above, the discomfort we have with the symptoms, and how they jar with what we know and hold dear, means that dementia demands exploration from Western writers. This theory is supported by the fact that existing fiction depicting dementia is predominantly from white, Western writers. We have tried to redress this by widening the canon in this particular anthology.

Second, narrativising dementia involves certain challenges that are interesting for writers. Dementia can entail memory loss and difficulties with language, both of which are necessary for telling stories. As such, a paradox arises when penning a narrator or character with dementia, because storytelling requires recall, putting events into order and into words. The creative prospects of narrativising dementia enable writers to experiment with form and narrative structure. Although Jan dealt with the ethical dimension of writing fiction about dementia in the introduction to this book, it is worth mentioning here: creative writers are not bound to tell the truth – that is the nature of fiction. They are free to use their creative licence, to play with the words available to them. That said, it is important that fictional representations of a lived experience (especially one that is so difficult for many) are well researched, honest and offer some kind of 'truth'. So while fictional representations of dementia have a complex relation to reality and peoples' lived experiences, they work best when they speak to, represent and interrogate different aspects of the condition, as the range of stories held here do. In the sections that follow, I provide examples of how the writers in this collection use language creatively to represent experiences of dementia.

Missing words

Although not all forms of dementia bring language difficulties, my research found that fiction often depicts this symptom, perhaps because it allows writers to experiment with language and memory in their stories. There are different ways of doing this. A character with dementia might repeat parts of the story, with us re-reading it verbatim, feeling like we've been here before, just like Niamh's father repeats, 'I had a Merc, once,' in Chris Wright's 'Downbeat'. This gives us a sense of being caught in a loop, reliving the same memories on repeat.

Writers often depict the how characters with dementia can't find a specific word; if readers are experiencing the story from their perspective, we share in that loss and subsequent confusion. Of course, a story would not be readable if words were lost too often, or across whole sentences. Yet Anna Jean Hughes takes this technique to the limit in 'Sound Distraction', with opaque descriptions such as, 'She holds something out to me. It's orange round. Only small. I don't take it, so she starts to tear its skirt off.' Readers have to work hard to decipher that the character with dementia is describing a mandarin orange. First, the object is referred to using the unspecific term 'something', then by using the unusual word order in 'orange round' (noun + adjective), then by replacing the action of peeling its skin with a visually similar action 'tearing its skirt off'. This example illustrates how language can be used creatively to mirror the experience of dementia. The language lost to the character is also lost to the reader. The simple gesture of being offered a mandarin orange is made strange and alien, giving us insight into how dementia might affect daily experience. While there are many such examples across the stories in this collection, Anna Jean Hughes explores this to the utmost, offering a strange and profound simulation of the experience of dementia through word loss, word play and perceptual difficulties.

Although my research focused on fiction told from the perspective of characters with dementia, the contributions to this anthology are told from the perspectives of other characters too. Reading these contributions has made me realise that 'missing words' is not just an affliction attributed to characters with dementia. The narrator in Paul McVeigh's story, 'Coming and Going', describes his father as follows: 'Recently, someone's been there, just not the man who was my dad. A new man who bore no resemblance to the Dad I knew, physically or in personality. My not-dad.' Here, it is not the person *with* dementia, but the person *observing* it who uses under-specific terms: 'someone' and 'a new man'. This made me appreciate how dementia is also a new experience for the loved one, who can struggle to come to terms with the changing identity of a parent.

Interestingly, even the word 'dementia' is avoided entirely in some of the stories in this collection, where instead the symptoms or changes are called 'his *illness*', ('My Way Home', Caleb Azumah Nelson), or 'a *waywardness* in Mam' ('This Small Giddy Life', Nuala O'Connor), or 'her mother's *condition*' ('Heatwave', Oona Frawley). The avoidance of the term 'dementia' in these stories might reflect the characters' experience of the 'unknown', of the symptoms pre-diagnosis, or even a discomfort with the label itself. This technique captures how verbalising dementia, whether a character is living through it or watching a loved one, is difficult. As Henrietta McKervey's narrator observes in 'A New Day, Tomorrow', 'I'd use other words if I had them, but I don't. Language is like that. It lets you down when you need it most.' Yet these stories still capture what it feels like to grapple for words, when our experience is hard to understand and express.

The present, the body and the senses

My research found that fiction about dementia tends to focus on the body and bodily experience in the here and now. Most of the stories in this collection are told in the present tense; this is not the norm for fiction, but corresponds with what I've seen in fiction about dementia. I think the present tense allows writers to depict how dementia demands living in the moment, and emphasises the importance of sensory and emotive experience over memory. When using the present tense, writers are more free to explore present experience, which is governed by immediate sensory descriptions and fleeting emotions. I found these often go hand in hand, as in this example from Suad Aldarra's 'The Three Strangers': 'My heartbeats slow down like the end of a song. I am safe now.' The first sentence describes a physical sensation; the second, an emotion, and we are invited to make an association between the two. I believe that fiction is uniquely placed to capture sensory and emotive experience in this way (can you imagine a hospital pamphlet doing the same?!). I also believe that this technique reminds us of what might be important in dementia care and interactions; that is, focusing on the present, on stimulating and supporting the senses and emotional wellbeing.

The body, behaviours and emotions of characters with dementia are sometimes filtered through the perspectives of other characters. Considering how this is done can reveal something about how dementia is viewed and understood from the outside looking in. In Chris Wright's 'Downbeat', Niamh describes her father:

> Dad was fast asleep on the sofa. His bony hand sat curled on top of his chest, rising and falling with the sway of

> *his shallow breath. Thick skin bunched and hung at the*
> *knuckles, his flesh spotted, pitted and lined in blue veins*
> *like a confluence on a map.*

This description focuses on his body in a vulnerable state, marked with age. No doubt it reflects the complex experience of observing a parent change physically, the role reversal of caring for a person who once cared for you. Earlier in the same story Niamh attempts to fulfil her new role, offering her father a nutritional shake:

> *I'm not fallin' fer that, he said, dropping his cigarette in*
> *the shake with a plop and a fizz and grinning at her*
> *through broken-grate teeth.*
>   *Fuck's sake, Dad.*

Despite his weak physical state and developing dementia, Niamh's father resists her care, dismissing it as trickery and literally putting out his cigarette in it. While this is immensely frustrating for his daughter, the interaction gives a sense of the tension between dementia, the ageing body, and an ongoing sense of agency in the person living through it. In this way, fiction can explore – without necessarily prescribing any answers – what it is like to live through these changes, and to observe them in a loved one. Characters with dementia can be shown to retain their 'personhood' through strong, defiant interactions such as this. Sometimes it is difficult to know if a person's behaviour is down to the dementia or is part of who they always were. For instance, Mary Morrissy's narrator in 'Fingerpost' is hurt by her friend's words and wonders, 'Was this the illness talking? Or was this what Delma had felt all along? In the past she'd often been sharpish with a hard glittery edge; now she was a sword unsheathed.' As this example shows, it can be hard to separate the person from the illness.

Alternatively, the effect of dementia on a person's character might be an unexpectedly positive one, as in Sinéad Gleeson's story, 'Immurement', where the affected mother develops a 'new late-stage sentimentality', not present pre-dementia, and manifesting in uncharacteristic tears. In Nuala O'Connor's story, 'This Small Giddy Life', 'There is awe and joy in her face, and it strikes me she is becalmed, no more the rushing hawk of her younger years. Stillness suits her, makes her cheerier, a thing none of us would ever have believed.' In these examples, daughters observe the effects of dementia as physical and behavioural changes in their mothers, in their bodies and faces. Their mothers may be losing memories and words, but consequently, they are experiencing the world in a more immediate and sensual way, which might facilitate a different kind of emotional connection with loved ones.

Metaphors

For many people, literary language means metaphors. But metaphors are a lot more commonplace, and central to the way we think, than you might imagine. Metaphorical language includes metaphors and their sisters, similes; both describe one thing in terms of another. Often, a metaphor or simile describes something that is quite abstract, or difficult to 'pin down', in terms of something more real or concrete. Although literary language is known for using creative metaphors, it often uses metaphors that are quite conventional and close to everyday ways of expressing things. For example, Sinéad Gleeson's narrator in 'Immurement' describes dementia as 'a burst pipe in the brain'. Thinking about our brains as plumbing systems might be helpful for understanding the physical changes brought by dementia. The brain, the mind and consciousness, all of which dementia can affect, are extremely difficult for us to describe, so metaphorical language can help.

The narrator of Caleb Azumah Nelson's story 'My Way Home', observes his father: 'His illness stays pressed to his chest, announces itself before he can announce himself, his agency lost somewhere in the swirl of memories he keeps trying to grasp.' The dementia ('his illness') is made physical, personified and given a voice that drowns out his father's, while the memories are also made physical and out of reach. Here, the metaphorical language helps the reader imagine the unnamed illness as a more tangible thing, and understand the son's perception of how it physically impacts upon his father. Our reading group research found that metaphors really strike readers and can shape or reinvent their perception of dementia.

Because it involves associations between concepts, metaphorical language reveals how we think. In everyday conversation, the brain is often talked about metaphorically as if it were an administrative or computer system. We can see this in fiction too, where the narrator of Henrietta McKervey's 'A New Day, Tomorrow' (who does not have dementia) describes 'the filing cabinets of my mind', where the brain is a filing system for our thoughts and memories. This is a useful shorthand for dealing with the brain and its complexities, but if applied to dementia, might invite a conceptualisation of the condition as one that corrupts the internal filing system, wiping the data. If our minds and 'processing power' are so closely aligned with our personhood, with our identity, then this conventional metaphor could lead to the assumption that losing 'data' (memory) is a loss of our identity, i.e. that dementia makes us less of a person. Metaphors, then, can smuggle powerful ways of thinking in language and shape the way that we think about the world and people around us.

Metaphorical language also has the power to *challenge* traditional ways of thinking, especially when it brings together unconventional concepts. For example, in 'The Three Strangers', Suad Aldarra uses a simile, 'I realised he was gone once again, like a beautiful sunset. I couldn't wait for him to rise again.' We don't often think of people as sunsets, that come and go with an infinite beauty. But doing so provides a comforting reassurance that this loved one will return and it will be a happy reunion. To be precise, it is not the narrator's *father* who is coming or going here, but his *consciousness*, so this example also offers a different way of understanding the human mind which, like a sunset, is universal and governed by nature. Like every individual consciousness, the sun will one day burn out, but the simile here conflates billions of years with a human lifetime – the duration doesn't matter; like the sun, we are all finite and life, while it lasts, is 'beautiful'.

Of course there are any number of ways that dementia, and our experience of it, can be represented in metaphorical language. But, hopefully, the examples discussed here illustrate how metaphorical language can help us handle difficult, invisible concepts such as dementia, help us understand them in more tangible ways, and even challenge or reshape our conventional ways of thinking about the experience.

Voices, perspectives and realities

There's something else that fiction can do, unlike any other kind of language. It can weave together voices and perspectives so that an event or experience can be understood in many different ways simultaneously. An extreme example of this trick is found in Naomi Krüger's 'People Who Want History, Want *History*'. Her 'story' is not a traditional narrative, instead it brings together fragments of different texts – care home documents, a transcribed interview, and a student's literature essay. Using these fragments, the reader has to piece together an understanding of the character with dementia and a young student's naïve interactions with him in a reminiscence session. The care home documents prescribe how to do 'reminiscence therapy' and how carers and therapists should interact with residents with dementia. The young student attempts to implement this guidance in a reminiscence session with Eddie, judiciously steering him away from 'sensitive' topics, such as gay sex and violence, by stuttering to tell a story, a Polish folktale. The folktale, retold in an extract from the student's university essay, is about memory, its loss and its trickery. As all these snippets are pieced together, we are shown a contrast between 'reminiscence' as the care home prescribes it and the student tries to implement it, and the way that Eddie, the lively character with dementia, prefers to do it. Eddie is not encumbered by the institutional regulations that govern the care home and the university student, so his speech comes across as more fluent, his interactions more confident and spirited. This story, a creative patchwork of different voices, makes us appreciate the communicative skills of people with dementia; their conversational contributions may not be orderly or conform to everyday norms and expectations, but they can be rich, impassioned and are worth listening to.

Fiction gives readers access to characters' speech and thoughts. In fact, access to other people's thoughts is one of the unique advantages of reading, one of the only ways of getting inside the mind of another person, and surely a big part of why we enjoy reading fiction. Writers can present the voices and thoughts of characters in different ways, allowing us readers to appreciate multiple perspectives on the same situation. This can be beneficial for our understanding of something like dementia, which affects different people in different ways. The following interaction is from 'Sound Distraction', by Anna Jean Hughes:

> *'Mams, where did you go?'*
> *It's my Pearl.*
> *'I'm here, girl'*

In this exchange, the narrator with dementia recognises and names her daughter 'Pearl' internally, even though she doesn't verbalise it. Instead, she calls her 'girl', leaving her daughter none the wiser that her mother, seemingly lost to her, recognises her by name. The reader has a privileged position, with insight into the mother's glimmer of recognition, but also a bittersweet awareness that the daughter doesn't know she was recognised. In this way, fiction can juxtapose different voices and perspectives, showing that the same situation is not experienced in the same ways by all those involved, and giving us a unique insight into the multiple experiences of dementia. The dramatic irony present here is something I found to be particularly pertinent in dementia fiction. If dementia entails a loss of memory, or an ability to express oneself, fiction provides a way of re-presenting those apparently 'lost' voices and thoughts. In this way, dementia fiction allows readers to understand the continued personhood of the character with dementia, even when it may not be visible to others.

We see a reversal of this in Elaine Feeney's story, 'What, You Egg', which is told from the perspective of a daughter who cares for her mother with advanced dementia. The daughter recounts her mother's early life spent by the Atlantic Ocean in Donegal but, unusually, does so using the second person, 'you': 'You love water … you've always wanted to jump in the sea.' This narrative technique creates an intimate dialogue between daughter and mother. But it also gives us a detailed account of the early life of the woman with dementia, at a time when she might not be able to verbalise it. In this way, narrative fiction can give voice to the voiceless. These fragments of her mother's past are interspersed with present-day interactions. In one, the daughter waits for her mother to come out of the shower, asking 'Are you swimming?', to which she responds, 'I am.' After the shower, her mother glows: 'I can't wait to tell her [Mrs Faye] I've been swimming in the mad ocean and that I was so happy.' This creates another kind of dramatic irony, where we readers know that the character with dementia is disorientated and understand that the daughter is facilitating her fantasy. Yet, through the mother's speech, we can see the joy the fantasy has brought her and understand the emotional benefits of the untruth. These examples show how fiction can narrate internal and external voices, leading readers to understand different perspectives and gain a multi-dimensional picture of how dementia can affect people.

As well as combining voices and perspectives in ways that other kinds of language cannot, fiction can also play with reality. The stories by Jan Carson and Caleb Klaces create alternative worlds to explore dementia, bending reality as we know it. While my research focused on fiction that represents dementia in a realistic way, these contributions offer something different. Klaces explores a world-within-a-world-within-a-world: a young man revisits his father's home, finds a story he wrote on an old computer, and tells that story, which is about using a portal to enter the mind and body of an older man called Brian. 'The Portal' is an experiment in what constitutes memory, reality and personhood, all of which dementia challenge. In 'Our Dear Ladies Have Outnumbered Us', Jan Carson's absurd reality is narrated by an unnamed collective, 'we', who run a care home for a bevy of characterful ladies. After the arrival of the enigmatic Angelica, who seems to lead the ladies astray, the power balance is disrupted and strange things start to happen. The alternative reality gives Jan a space to explore important issues in dementia care, such as power and agency, in an indirect and playful way.

It has been fascinating for me to observe how the contributions to this anthology correspond with my research on how dementia is represented in the minds of fictional characters. But the new stories collected here do a lot more than simply confirm my research findings. They add to the canon of dementia fiction by including a wider range of voices and perspectives than those previously published, giving a broader view of the experience. I hope to have shed some light on how creative language is uniquely placed to help readers understand dementia in ways that might facilitate awareness, understanding and care. Creative writing must be recognised as a form of cultural expression that allows key issues of our time, like dementia, to be interrogated and illuminated, with real-life consequence and value.

Acknowledgements

This anthology is the joyful culmination of several years of work and research. It arises from a research project, 'Dementia in the minds of characters and readers', led by Dr Jane Lugea (Queen's University Belfast) and generously funded by the Arts and Humanities Research Council (Project Reference: AH/S001476/1).

We are so grateful to everyone who contributed to both the anthology and the research project which inspired it. We'd like to extend our particular thanks to our wonderful research colleagues, Dr Gemma Carney, Dr Paula Devine and Dr Carolina Fernández-Quintanilla. You've been the most inspiring, encouraging and helpful people to work with. We couldn't have asked for a better team. The research project also benefitted greatly from the careful steer of our Advisory Panel, including Professor Tess Maginess, Professor Aagje Swinnen, Rachel McCance (Northern Ireland Museums Council) and staff from the Alzheimer's Society. We are particularly indebted to – and in awe of – everyone at Dementia NI. The staff and members provided invaluable insight into living with dementia and really helped to ensure these stories were both believable and urgent. You can find more about their incredible work at www.dementiani.org.

A huge heartfelt thank you to Aoife K. Walsh and the team at New Island including Susan McKeever, whose tireless work on the edit ensured each story packs a real punch. Thank you so much for bringing our creative vision to life and seeing the potential in this book. Thank you also to each of our wonderful writers who entered into the project with imagination and enthusiasm. You've been an absolute dream to work with and we can't wait to see what you do next. Finally, and most importantly, thank you to all the readers who've picked up this anthology. We hope it will leave you captivated, entertained and perhaps a little more aware of what it's like to live with dementia.

Contributors' Biographies

Suad Aldarra is a Syrian-Irish writer, public speaker and data scientist based in Dublin. She was selected as the Common Currency writer in residence for Cúirt International Festival and English/Irish PEN in 2021 and was awarded the Art Councils of Ireland English Literature bursary. Her debut memoir, *I Don't Want to Talk About Home*, was published by Doubleday Ireland in July 2022.

Caleb Azumah Nelson is a British-Ghanaian writer and photographer who currently lives in South East London. He was shortlisted for the BBC National Short Story Award 2020 for his story 'Pray'. He was selected by *The Observer* as one of the '10 best debut novelists of 2021'. His debut novel, *Open Water*, was published by Viking (UK) in February 2021 and by Grove Atlantic (US) in spring 2021. It has since been longlisted for the Desmond Elliott prize and the Gordon Burn prize, shortlisted for the Waterstones Book of the Year 2021 and the Dylan Thomas Prize 2022, and won the Costa First Novel Award 2021. In February 2022 *Open Water* was Waterstones Paperback of the Month.

Jan Carson is a writer and community arts facilitator based in Belfast. She has written a novel, *Malcolm Orange Disappears*, and a short story collection, *Children's Children*, both published by Liberties Press. She also wrote two micro-fiction collections, *Postcard Stories 1* and *2* (Emma Press) and a short story collection, *The Last Resort* (Doubleday). Her novel *The Fire Starters* (Doubleday) won the EU Prize for Literature for Ireland 2019. Jan's latest novel, *The Raptures* was published by Doubleday in early 2022.

Elaine Feeney has published three poetry collections. Her debut novel *As You Were* (Vintage) won The Kate O'Brien Prize, Dalkey Book Festival's Emerging Writer Prize and Society of Authors' McKitterick Prize. It was also shortlisted for the Rathbones-Folio Prize. She lectures at The National University of Ireland, Galway. Her novel, *How to Build a Boat* will be published in 2023.

Oona Frawley was born in New York to Irish actor parents and is associate professor of English at Maynooth University. Her novel, *Flight*, was published in 2014 by Tramp Press, and her creative work appears most recently in *Banshee Magazine*. She is currently working on a book project of creative non-fiction.

Sinéad Gleeson's essay collection *Constellations* won Non-Fiction Book of the Year at the 2019 Irish Book Awards and the Dalkey Literary Award for Emerging Writer. Her short stories have appeared in *Being Various* (Faber) and *Repeal the 8th* (Unbound). She has edited five anthologies, most recently *This Woman's Work: Essays on Music* with Kim Gordon. She is working on a novel.

Anna Jean Hughes is a writer and editor living in London.

Caleb Klaces's most recent books are the poetry collection *Away From Me* and *Fatherhood,* a novel, both published by Prototype. He teaches at York Centre for Writing, York St John University.

Naomi Krüger is a short story writer and novelist. Her first novel, *May* (Seren, 2018) is partly narrated by a character with dementia and explores both the difficulties of memory, and the possibilities of connection. She is a senior lecturer in Literature and Creative Writing at the University of Central Lancashire.

Dr **Jane Lugea** is Senior Lecturer in English Language at Queen's University Belfast. She is interested in language use and linguistic creativity. As Principal Investigator on the AHRC-funded 'Dementia in the minds of characters and readers project', she led an interdisciplinary team exploring how dementia is represented in the minds of fictional characters, and how readers respond to them. This project revealed the capacity for fictional representations of dementia to increase awareness and understanding towards lived experiences of the condition. Jane is author of *World Building in Spanish and English Spoken Narratives* (Bloomsbury, 2016) and co-author *of Stylistics: Text, Cognition and Corpus* (Palgrave Macmillan, forthcoming).

Henrietta McKervey has published four critically acclaimed novels; *A Talented Man, Violet Hill, The Heart of Everything* and *What Becomes of Us*. She holds a Hennessy First Fiction Award and won the inaugural UCD Maeve Binchy Travel Award. She is a regular contributor to the *Irish Independent* and RTÉ radio. She is originally from Belfast and lives in Dublin.

Paul McVeigh's debut novel, *The Good Son*, won The Polari First Novel Prize, The McCrea Literary Award and was shortlisted for many others including the Prix de Roman Cezam. His short stories have appeared in *The Irish Times*, *The London Magazine* and *The Stinging Fly*, as well as on BBC Radio 3, 4 & 5, and Sky Arts. His writing has been translated into seven languages.

Mary Morrissy is the author of three novels, *Mother of Pearl*, *The Pretender* and *The Rising of Bella Casey*, and two collections of stories, *A Lazy Eye* and *Prosperity Drive*. A fourth novel, *Penelope Unbound*, is forthcoming in 2023. Her work has won her the Hennessy Prize and a Lannan Foundation Award. A member of Aosdána, she is a journalist and teacher of creative writing.

Nuala O'Connor's fifth novel, *Nora*, about Nora Barnacle and James Joyce, was a Top 10 historical novel in *The New York Times* and the One Dublin One Book choice for 2022. Nuala curated –*Love, says Bloom*, an exhibition about the Joyce family, at the Museum of Literature Ireland (MOLI). She is editor at flash fiction e-journal *Splonk*.

Chris Wright is a fiction writer from Bangor, Northern Ireland. He has been longlisted for the Irish Book Awards Short Story of the Year, was runner-up in The Mairtín Crawford Award, and his work has featured in several print anthologies and publications. Chris is currently studying for an MA in Creative Writing at Queen's University, Belfast.